How to be
to be
Pre-Med

How to be Pre-Med

A Harvard MD's
Medical School Preparation Guide
for Students and Parents

Suzanne M. Miller, MD

info@MDadmit.com
www.MDadmit.com

The prices and rates stated in this book are subject to change.

Library of Congress Control Number: 2013902048

ISBN: 978-1-936633-55-5

Cover design by Casey Hooper
Layout design by Lori Lynch
Text set in Galliard

Printed in the United States of America

To Adam, my greatest love and biggest fan.

Acknowledgements

I would like to thank the pre-meds I have met though my medical school advising journey, who have spurred this book's creation, built MDadmit from an idea to a leading company, and reminded me of why I became a physician. I am proud of you all.

Thanks to Sharon Miller for her editing genius, Casey Hooper for cover design, Lori Lynch for layout design, Dennis Kunimura for graphical work, and all of the pre-meds who gave permission to reference their work.

Also by Dr. Suzanne M. Miller

The Medical School Admissions Guide: A Harvard MD's
Week-by-Week Admissions Handbook, 2nd Edition

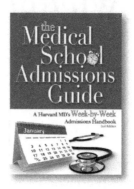

Available at amazon.com, barnesandnoble.com, and MDadmit.com

How To Get Into Medical School With A Low GPA

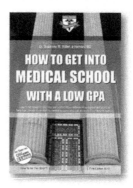

Available at howtobepremed.com

Contents

Who Should Read This Book

xi

A Note to Parents

xiii

Preface

xv

Acronyms

xxi

Bucket 1: Academics

1

Bucket 2: Research

35

Bucket 3: Community Service

53

Bucket 4: Extracurriculars

79

Bucket 5: Clinical Experience

91

Bucket 6: Application Skills

99

Who Should Read This Book

How To Be Pre-Med assists high school, college, and non-traditional students interested in becoming physicians by describing the pre-med route from start to finish using the Six Buckets model I developed through over a decade of medical school admissions advising. This guide is equally helpful to those hoping to pursue a medical career and to loved ones, such as parents, spouses, relatives, and friends, supporting a pre-med.

I created How to be Pre-Med to serve as a prequel to the best-selling The Medical School Admissions Guide: A Harvard MD's Week-by-Week Admissions Handbook because readers frequently provided feedback wishing they had received similar expert guidance sooner in the pre-med process.

How To Be Pre-Med covers all information required to excel

as a pre-med and prepare for the medical school application process. I suggest you read this book as soon as you decide to pursue the pre-med path to help strategize selection of undergraduate or post-baccalaureate experiences. Then return to it each year to assess how you are filling up the Six Buckets.

Once you have decided to apply to medical school, pick up the latest edition of The *Medical School Admissions Guide* and follow the weekly steps required to create the best application possible to maximize your chances of admission.

A Note to Parents

Over the past decade as a Harvard pre-med tutor and then as CEO of MDadmit medical school admissions consulting, I have witnessed how parenting a pre-med can be just as stressful as being a pre-med. Parents of students who want to be doctors often struggle with supporting their child during the complex pre-med and medical school application processes without seeming overbearing.

You may feel overwhelmed by the pre-med academic, research, community service, extracurricular, clinical, and application requirements. Perhaps you are frustrated by the lack of personalized advising provided by your child's undergraduate institution where advisors often serve hundreds of applicants. Maybe you don't know which of the Internet's conflicting advice to believe. Or possibly you applied to medical school years ago and are uncertain how the process has changed.

Being a pre-med parent is certainly difficult. But you have found the best way to help – arm yourself with knowledge of how the process works. I suggest you read *How to be Pre-Med* yourself, and then hand it to your pre-med. After one read of this guide, you will know more about being pre-med than any parent on the block (and many admissions advisors).

Preface

The Calling

Welcome as you start the journey to becoming a physician. Despite the grumbling you may hear from physicians and the media about bureaucratic red tape and our "broken" healthcare system, doctoring is still a wonderful profession. Physicians help others in a tangible way on a daily basis and possess portable skills useful throughout the world. Being a doctor is more of a calling or a vocation than a job, and it can be a very satisfying career.

That being said, the medical profession involves great personal and economic sacrifices. To become a practicing physician in the United States requires four years of undergraduate school, four more years of medical school, three to seven years of post-graduate residency training, and often two to three more years of fellowship training. Most doctors do not start their careers as independent physicians and begin earning a decent wage until age 30 or later. Going down the medicine path is not for everyone. In fact, I always give the same advice to those considering becoming a physician: If you will be happy pursuing any profession other than medicine, go do that. If not, become a doctor.

There is no need to rush the decision to become a physician. Interestingly, the American Association of Medical Colleges (AAMC) gathered data on when medical school matriculating students knew they wanted to be doctors. Here are the results:

- Before high school: 20%
- During high school or before college: 29%
- During the first two years of college: 24%
- During junior year of college: 11%
- During senior year of college: 4%
- After receiving bachelor's degree: 10%
- After receiving advanced degree: 2%

(Source: AAMC's 2011 Matriculating Student Questionnaire – https://www.aamc.org/data/msq/)

Based on the AAMC data, it is quite common to decide on medicine as a career during or after college. Thus, I have written this book to be relevant for all pre-meds, whether you make the decision to become a doctor in high school or 10 years into another profession. I have known many individuals who left the pre-med track during college, pursued another career, and returned to pre-med courses years later because the nagging desire to become a doctor persisted. If you have the calling to be a physician, it is highly likely you will eventually become one.

The Buckets

Once you have heard the call to doctorhood, you will be entering a complex and competitive pre-med environment. To help navigate the often-stressful pre-med process, I developed the Six Buckets model used in this book. These Six Buckets include:

 Academics

 Research

 Community Service

 Extracurriculars

 Clinical Experience

 Application Skills

Each bucket represents a critical component of the pre-med process. Please note the Six Buckets should not be used as a checklist. You can't simply perform an activity from each bucket for a few weeks and expect to get into medical school. The purpose of the Six Buckets is to serve as an overarching guide to help plan how to spend your time. As you will see, some activities can fill multiple buckets. Some of your buckets may end up more filled than others. But no bucket should be left empty. As with all things in life, being pre-med and getting into medical school is not about checking the boxes; it's about doing what you love and doing it well.

I consider myself successful if you walk away from this book with the following themes tucked under your belt:

- Only become a doctor if you can think of doing nothing else
- Don't just check the boxes
- If you do what you love, you will do it well
- Getting into medical school requires telling a compelling story

Good luck, get going, and get in!

—Dr. Miller

Legal Disclaimer

I certainly cannot guarantee you success as a pre-med and admission to medical school by reading this book and following its advice. But I can assure your pre-med path will be less stressful and chances of medical school admission success will improve by learning the details of "how to be pre-med."

The author/publisher of this book has used her best efforts in preparing this book. The author/publisher makes no representation or warranties with respect to the accuracy, applicability, fitness, or completeness of the contents of this book. The information contained in this book is strictly for educational purposes. Therefore, if you wish to apply ideas contained in this book, you are taking full responsibility for your actions. The author/publisher shall in no event be held liable to any party for any direct, indirect, punitive, special, incidental, or other consequential damages arising directly or indirectly from any use of this material, which is provided "as is" and without warranties.

The author/publisher does not warrant the performance, effectiveness, or applicability of any websites listed in this book. All websites are listed for information purposes only and are not warranted for content, accuracy, or any other implied or explicit purpose.

The author/publisher of this book made every effort to be as accurate and complete as possible in the creation of the book's content. However, due to the rapidly changing nature of medical school admissions, she does not warrant or represent at any time that the contents within are accurate. Application fees, dates, deadlines, websites, and addresses, in addition to admissions requirements, change every year, and it is the reader's responsibility to stay up-to-date on such changes.

The author/publisher will not be responsible for any losses or damages of any kind incurred by the reader whether directly or indirectly arising from the use of the information found in this book.

Acronyms

The pre-med process and this book are full of acronyms. I have put them all in one place for easy reference.

AMCAS	American Medical College Application Service
TMDSAS	Texas Medical & Dental Schools Application Service
OMSAS	Ontario Medical Schools Application Service
AACOMAS	American Association of Colleges of Osteopathic Medicine Application Service
AAMC	Association of American Medical Colleges
AACOM	American Association of Colleges of Osteopathic Medicine
MCAT	Medical College Admission Test
FAP	Fee Assistant Program
MD	Doctor of Medicine
DO	Doctor of Osteopathy

MBA	Master of Business Administration
JD	Juris Doctor (Law)
MPH	Master of Public Health
MPA	Master of Public Administration
PhD	Doctor of Philosophy
USMLE	United States Medical Licensing Examination

CHAPTER 1

Academics

As you well know, academics are a huge part of the medical school admissions process. Academics are important, no doubt, but I often see pre-meds who put too much emphasis on academics to the detriment of other parts of their applications. I like to think of academics as a hurdle you have to cross in order to be considered for medical school admissions. Once your pass the bar, you can move on to the often more interesting parts of your life such as research, community service, extracurricular, and clinical activities.

Major

"Pre-med" is not a major. It is a designation used to define students taking the required courses for entry into medical school. You can major in anything you'd like in college as long as you take the necessary classes (see below for list of required courses). There is no need to major in a science. In fact, humanities majors often do very well in medical school admissions because of their well-rounded background. I concentrated in a form of history in college and took pre-med courses as electives. There is no one major that will guarantee you admission to medical school. The key is to focus on taking classes in subjects that excite you and you can't wait to get home and read about. When you are passionate about a subject, you will likely excel in it.

If you do decide to major in a non-science subject and want to go straight to medical school after college, it is important to plan in advance to be sure you can fit all major, core, and pre-med coursework into the allotted undergraduate timeframe. But do know there is no rule stating you have to complete all pre-med classes during undergraduate years. You can always take time off after college to complete the pre-med requirements. In fact, you do not have to take one pre-med course as an undergraduate if you so choose. Post-baccalaureate programs have been set up throughout the country offering pre-med coursework either over an intensive one-year period or part-time over multiple years. You can find the details of such programs in a searchable database maintained by the Association of American Medical Colleges (AAMC): http://services.aamc.org/postbac/. In summary, feel free to major in visual arts or government or literature as long as you have a plan for how to complete the pre-med courses during or after college.

Courses

The academic requirements of medical school admissions are relatively simple. The necessary courses are laid out in the *Medical School Academic Requirements* (MSAR) published yearly by AAMC.

The MSAR is a must-have resource for any pre-med as it not only lists the requirements but also gives specific demographics of each school, including location, class size, gender and race percentages, and average GPA/Medical College Admission Test (MCAT) scores. The AAMC recently started a new website (https://services.aamc.org/30/msar/home) offering some MSAR information for free and charging for access to the full database. I strongly suggest you buy the MSAR to obtain the full data set.

Everyone applying to medical school must complete the following courses:

PRE-MED COURSE REQUIREMENTS

Course	Number of Semesters	Semester Hours	Lab Required?	Comments
Biology	2	8	Yes	1 semester with strong genetics component
Inorganic Chemistry	2	8	Yes	
Organic Chemistry	2	8	Yes	
Physics	2	8	Yes	
English	2	8	No	Most schools want strong writing component
Math	2	8	No	Most schools want calculus level courses

Based on these medical school requisites, the acronym BCPM (biology, chemistry, physics, math) has emerged to describe the science-oriented requirements. Certain medical schools have other course requirements beyond those listed above. One semester of biochemistry is the most common additional required course. As you'll see in the MSAR, most schools merely "suggest" instead of "require" a whole gaggle of classes including:

- Behavioral Sciences
- Zoology
- Computer Science
- Genetics
- Psychology
- Social sciences
- Statistics

With a new MCAT arriving in 2015 emphasizing social and behavioral science, many medical schools are strongly suggesting pre-meds take psychology and sociology. See the MCAT section below for a discussion of the current MCAT exam and future changes.

Looking at these requirements, you can see how it is possible to be a humanities major and a pre-med. If you lay out your classes carefully ahead of time, you can pursue virtually any major and still fit in the pre-med coursework.

When choosing courses, it is important to know how the medical school application will categorize your classes. Fortunately, AAMC has prepared a "Course Classification Guide" (https://www.aamc.org/students/download/181694/data/amcas_course_classification_guide.pdf) laying out exactly how your courses will be categorized. Consult this document early to ensure the course you think will "count" for the pre-med requirements actually does count. Let's say you want to take a pharmacology class and expect it to fulfill the biology or chemistry portion of your pre-med requirements. According to the "Course Classification Guide," a pharmacology class will not be considered a "BCPM" course and, thus, likely will not satisfy the pre-med requirements according to most medical schools. Of course, you can still take the class. But knowing it won't fulfill a pre-med requirement will help you plan other courses and ensure you have time and energy to complete all pre-requisites.

I am often asked how important it is to take upper level classes to satisfy the pre-med requirements. If you can get A's in harder classes, then I suggest you go for it. But a B in an upper level class looks worse to the medical school admissions committees than an A in an intro course. Medical school admissions committee members don't have the time to memorize the level of each class at every college or university. It is much easier to sift through applications by looking at a total grade point average (GPA) than to weigh grades earned in upper level classes more than those earned in lower level courses. My suggestion is to challenge yourself as much as possible in your coursework without sacrificing GPA.

GPA

Often analyzed together with the MCAT, the GPA tells medical school admissions committees whether or not you can handle rigorous medical school coursework. Medical school admissions committees look at three different GPAs – cumulative GPA (total GPA), science GPA (BCPM – biology, chemistry, physics, and math), and all other GPA (AO, everything except BCPM). Most admissions committees look first at the cumulative GPA, and then confirm the science GPA is not far off that total mark. In general, most applicants have a slightly lower science GPA than total GPA. For the purposes of this book, I will discuss total GPA.

The medical school application requires you to enter coursework information and grades from all post-secondary schools you have attended. This includes community college, four-year undergraduate, study abroad, and graduate classes. In other words, you can't hide a C earned in the underwater basket weaving course taken as a lark while studying abroad. Given every course you take after high school goes on your application, please choose each class carefully. Feel free to take an unusual class of particular interest to you, but know the grade you earn in every course "counts" towards your GPA for medical school admissions.

Here is the most frequent pre-med question: "What GPA will get me into medical school?" Unfortunately, there is no clear-cut answer. Many think it takes a 4.0 GPA to gain acceptance to medical school. They are wrong. Pre-meds with 4.0 GPAs have used my consulting services after medical schools rejected them. Sure, you generally need good grades to get into medical school, but there is no exact GPA that guarantees admission. Medical school admissions committees look at each pre-med's "whole package" when deciding who gets into medical school. Great grades are not enough to secure admission. Did you notice academics are only one of this book's Six Buckets?

When describing the role of GPA in the medical school admissions process, I like to use a hurdle analogy. Once you have passed the academic GPA bar set by admissions committees, the rest of your application then becomes more important. Jump over the GPA hurdle and continue down the track to other significant and often more interesting items such as your personal experiences, life goals, and character. You may wonder exactly where the GPA bar is set. Interestingly, the GPA level depends on many factors and is set at different heights for different applicants.

In addition to each medical school setting a different GPA bar, the GPA hurdle height also moves depending on your race, gender, age, disadvantaged status, undergraduate institution, major, state of legal residence, and life experiences. In general, I suggest a 3.0 GPA is the lowest viable GPA for US medical school admissions. Do some applicants with 2.9 GPAs get into medical school? Yes. But this is very rare and usually involves extreme and unusual circumstances.

What is a "safe" GPA level? Achieve a 3.7 GPA or higher and you likely don't have to fear GPA holding you back in medical school admissions. Of course, this doesn't mean a 3.7 GPA is enough to get you into medical school. An applicant with a 3.7 GPA and a 25 MCAT likely won't be accepted. In addition, a pre-med with a 3.7 GPA, 37 MCAT, and no clinical experience likely will not gain admission. Medical school admissions committees are looking for the whole package, including your academic, research, community service, extracurricular, and clinical experience.

Let's look at the most recent data published by the AAMC (www.aamc.org) that reveals how GPA hurdle height changes based on different schools and applicant characteristics. Each graph on the following pages plots mean GPAs. Of course, by definition, an average GPA statistic is not perfect as most pre-meds who make up the mean scored either lower or higher than the mean. But the average GPA does give you a general sense of where you need to be GPA-wise to gain admission. In addition, the GPA trends based on private medical schools, public medical schools, state of legal residence, race/ethnicity, gender, and undergraduate major reveal how different medical schools have different GPA bars and how certain characteristics affect your chances of admissions based on GPA numbers.

How to Be Pre-Med

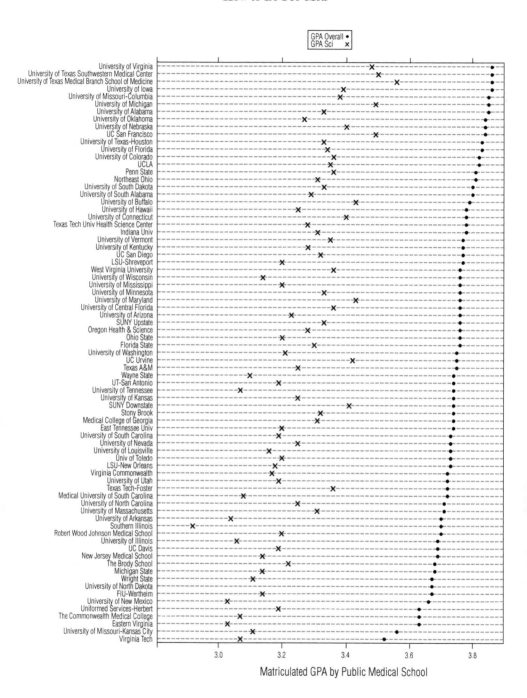

Matriculated GPA by Public Medical School

Academics

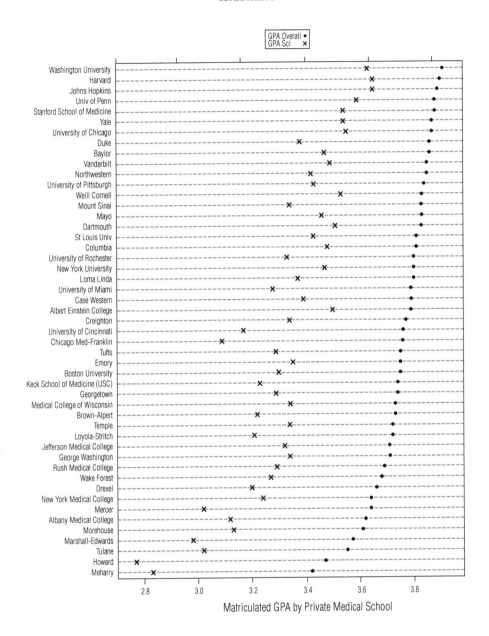

Matriculated GPA by Private Medical School

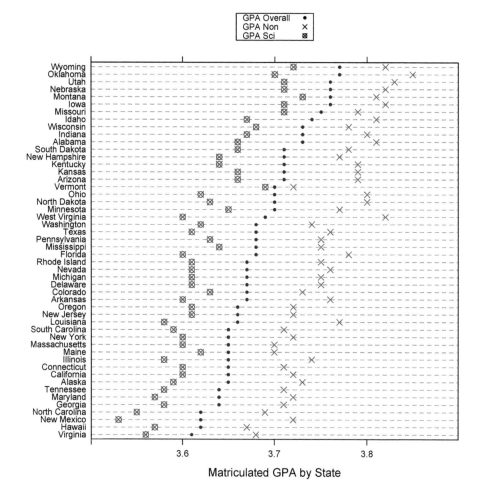

Matriculated GPA by State

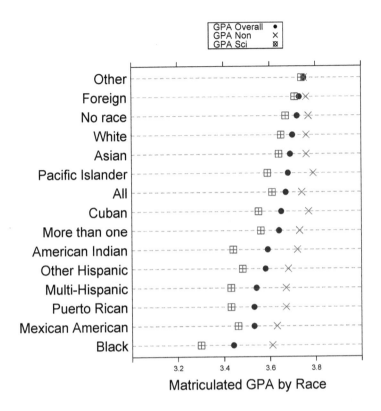

Matriculated GPA by Race

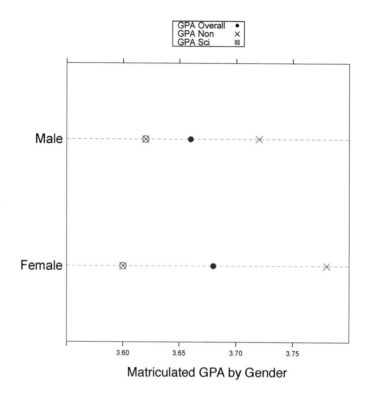

Matriculated GPA by Gender

Academics

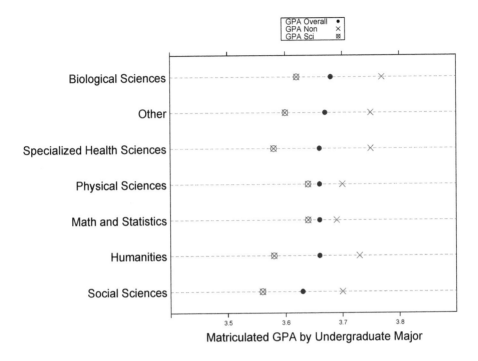

Matriculated GPA by Undergraduate Major

Isn't the data fascinating? It proves my point that each pre-med does not have the same GPA hurdle to cross because the GPA bar moves depending on certain characteristics. Medical school admissions committees certainly do not want to admit it, but as you can see from the medical school admissions data, the GPA bar is set at different heights for different groups. I don't want to offend anyone with my overt discussions of these qualities, but the medical school admissions data tells the story. There are certain characteristics that give a pre-med an advantage in the medical school admissions process such as living in certain state, being born a racial or ethnic minority, or studying the humanities. Some of these qualities you have no control over. Others you can influence. My goal here is not to discuss the fairness of the admissions process, but to make the process as transparent as possible for you. By understanding what category the medical school admissions committees will put you into, you will be a better pre-med.

Let's dive deeper into the AAMC data. The mean GPA for public medical schools in the US ranges from 3.5 to 3.9 and for private schools ranges from 3.4 to 3.9. This doesn't mean, however, that as a Virginia resident you will likely gain acceptance to the University of New Mexico with a 3.5 GPA. Public schools, also known as "state" schools, give a strong preference to in-state applicants because these applicants or their parents pay state income taxes. Unless you are an outstanding candidate, it is extremely difficult to get into an out-of-state school. When applying to medical school, you should generally focus on your own state school(s) and private schools where you fit into the GPA range. And if you reside in a state on the lower end of the mean GPA range, like Virginia or Hawaii, then you are fortunate.

When it comes to race and gender, the AAMC data shows

certain ethnic minorities, including Black, Hispanic, and American Indian applicants, have lower mean GPAs than Asian, White, and Foreign applicants, while men and women have similar average GPAs. The average science GPA is a bit lower and average non-science GPA a tad higher for women compared to men. Interestingly, women used to have an advantage in medical school admissions because fewer women then men applied. Now, more women than men are both applying and matriculating to medical school. With more women applying to medical school but more men working as physicians, an applicant's gender has little bearing on medical school admissions.

Age and disadvantaged status information is not provided by the AAMC but these characteristics do play a role in how admissions committees categorize your application and view the GPA. In general, most medical school applicants apply directly from college or take one to two years off. However, it is not uncommon for applicants to be in their late 20s and 30s. I have had clients in their 40s get into medical school. There is no absolute age cut off for medical school admissions. If you are on the older side, you will have the advantages of maturity and years of experience but the added burden of proving to admissions committees why you want to leave your current career to attend medical school. Disadvantaged status plays a large role in medical school admissions. Schools leave the definition of "disadvantaged" up to each applicant. To be considered for disadvantaged status, you must write an extra essay for the application explaining exactly why you have been underprivileged or overcome an extreme barrier. Though economic and race status are the most common reasons used to define "disadvantaged," other issues, such as family situations and personal illness, may be considered for disadvantaged status. Overcoming a disadvantage can put your GPA in a more positive light and often gives an advantage in medical school admissions.

When assessing GPA, medical schools will also look at your major and the strength of your educational institutions. Most pre-meds are science majors. Thus, being a humanities major gives you a slight advantage when it comes to medical school admissions. And, as you can see in the AAMC data, humanities and social science majors have slightly lower mean GPAs than biology majors. With regards to alma maters, reputation matters. A 3.5 from a top-tier institution will carry more weight than from a community college. Given the cost of private colleges in the US, it is completely understandable why one would want to pursue a community college or local public school post-secondary education. But if you do follow one of these paths, know the GPA bar you have to cross may be higher when compared to pre-meds from top 20 schools.

I don't want you to think that because you fit into an ethnic or racial minority category or come from a disadvantaged background or live in a state with a comparatively low mean GPA that you don't have to worry about academic performance. This could not be further from the truth. GPA is an important criterion used by medical schools admissions committees to evaluate whether any applicant, regardless of background, can handle the academic rigor of medical school.

If you underperform as a pre-med, however, all hope of becoming a physician is not lost. Dealing with a low GPA in the medical school admissions process is tough and hopefully you will not be in this situation. But if you are a pre-med with a low GPA, I have created a separate e-book just for you. *How To Get Into Medical School With A Low GPA* (http://www.howtobepremed.com/how-to-get-into-medical-school-with-a-low-gpa) provides a framework for how applicants should approach their particular low GPA situations, offers specific mitigation strategies drawn from true-to-life experiences of past clients, and presents personal statements from applicants who got into medical school with a low GPA.

MCAT

In addition to completing pre-med coursework, anyone applying to US medical schools needs to take the Medical College Admissions Test (MCAT). The test is run by the AAMC and used by medical school admissions committees along with your GPA to determine if you can handle medical school academics. The 2013 MCAT exam is slightly changed from previous years and a completely new test will emerge in 2015. I discuss both the current exam and the expected 2015 changes below.

MCAT Essentials

As of 2013, the MCAT exam only consists of three official sections because the writing sample has been removed and replaced with a voluntary trial section to test questions for the new 2015 exam. Those who participate in the trial section receive a $30 Amazon gift card. The 2013 and 2014 exams will have four parts:

- Physical Sciences (PS)
- Verbal Reasoning (VR)
- Biological Sciences (BS)
- Trial Section (TS)

Some important MCAT facts:

- The test is a little over five hours long including breaks. Total content time is approximately four hours and five minutes.
- The test is self-paced (*i.e.*, you choose when to take a break) but each section has a time limit.
- You are able to review and change answers within a section until you reach the time limit for that particular section. Unfortunately, once you have completed a section, you cannot go back and change answers.
- You may make notations on the screen such as highlighting a passage or striking out an answer choice.
- Scores will be available in approximately 30 days after exam completion. Scores are sent directly to AMCAS. Be sure to select sending scores to your pre-med advisor as well (it's free).
- If you think you performed very poorly on the exam, you can cancel the score at the end of the test and it will be voided. There is no way to cancel the score once you leave the exam site.
- You may only take the MCAT three times in one year.
- MCAT scores expire in three years.

Here's a breakdown of the test sections, questions, and time limits from the AAMC's *2013 MCAT Essentials*, a free publications available as a pdf document at **www.aamc.com**.

TEST SECTION	QUESTIONS	TIME
Tutorial (optional)		10 minutes
Examinee Agreement		10 minutes
Physical Sciences	52	70 minutes
Break (optional)		10 minutes
Verbal Reasoning	40	60 minutes
Break (optional)		10 minutes
Biological Sciences	52	70 minutes
Void Question		5 minutes
Break (optional)		10 minutes
Trial Section (Optional)	32	45 minutes
Survey (optional)	12	10 minutes
Total Content Time		4 hours, 5 minutes
Total Seat Time		5 hours, 10 minutes

The PS, VR, and BS sections are scored on a scale of 15 (15 being the highest score possible). The trial section is not scored. You will see scores reported as:

PS 15 VR 15 BS 15 or 45

Most pre-meds take the MCAT in the spring prior to applying to medical school. If you want to go directly from undergraduate studies to medical school, you will have to sit the test in the spring of junior year at the latest. But lucky for you, the MCAT schedule has become more flexible in recent years and allows you to pick a date that best meets your personal schedule. In the old days (2006 and prior), the MCAT was a written exam offered twice a year in April and August. This meant almost everyone had to take the exam on one infamous day in April in order to receive scores in time to submit the primary medical school application, called the American Medical College Application Service (AMCAS), when it started accepting applications in June. Now, the MCAT is computer-based and offered on 25 different days spread out over the year. As of 2013, the exam is being offered in January, March, April, May, June, July, August, and September (https://www.aamc.org/students/applying/mcat/reserving/ 261800/deadlineandscorerelease.html). With these more flexible dates, you can now select a day that best fits your study habits and overall admissions timeline. In general, regular and late MCAT registrations close two weeks and one week prior to the exam, respectively.

For exact details on exam times and registration requirements, visit www.aamc.org/mcat. Testing locations can be found at http:// services.aamc.org/20/mcat/sitelisting. To officially register and check for updated information, see https://www.aamc.org/students/applying /mcat/reserving/. Regular registration for the MCAT costs $270. Late registration is an additional $75 and rescheduling a date or changing your test center costs $90 more. Discounts are available for individuals who qualify for the AAMC's Fee Assistance Program – see https://www.aamc.org/students/applying/fap/ for details.

Things to consider when setting your MCAT test date:

- Will I take a MCAT class or online course?
- When will my class or job schedule allow sufficient study time?
- Will I forget material just learned in classes if I put off taking the exam?
- Will I get my test score back in time to submit the AMCAS application early in the application cycle? (AMCAS opens in early June.)

- Will I definitely apply to medical school this cycle? (The MCAT score expires after three years.)
- If I bomb the exam, will I have enough time to retake it? (Be aware that many MCAT sites fill up, and it may be impossible to retake the test unless someone drops a reservation.)
- Will I be most likely to perform my best on this test date? (You may only take the test three times per year.)

When preparing for the MCAT, have the mindset that you will only sit the test once. You should never go into the MCAT unprepared as a "practice" session because medical schools see every unexpired score. Many applicants wonder if they should retake the MCAT after a suboptimal performance. Generally speaking, you should only retest if you can improve your score by at least three points, which is quite hard to do. Good reasons for retaking the test include:

- You were not prepared (did not study well, had not taken the appropriate classes).
- You were sick as a dog on test day.
- You freaked out.
- Your score is very uneven and you strongly believe you can improve the low score (for example, PS 7 VR 11 BS 12 and you are confident you can improve the PS to 10).
- Your score is less than 30 and you strongly believe you can get it above 30 (ideally three or more points higher).

Remember, unless you cancel the score at the test site immediately after the exam, the admissions committees will see every unexpired MCAT score you have earned. MCAT scores expire after three years and you may take the test only three times in a given year. The AAMC did a survey of medical school admissions committees to see how they use multiple MCAT scores. The survey revealed several methods. Some schools view all scores equally and look for improvement. Others look only at the most recent score. Some average all scores. Still others take the highest score. Of these four methods, the first is most common.

Similar to the GPA, no one MCAT score guarantees admission to medical school. But data compiled by the AAMC shows applicants with scores in each section of >10 are more likely to be accepted. Based on this data and my personal experience with medical school admissions, I view a 30 as the minimum MCAT score required to get into a US allopathic medical school. Be aware, the verbal reasoning score is just as important as the science section scores. Why? Because data shows a pre-med's performance on the verbal reasoning section of the MCAT directly correlates with his or her United States Medical Licensing Examination (USMLE) Step 1 board score taken in medical school. Medical schools care very much about your likelihood of passing the USMLE as the schools are often judged by their students' pass rate.

Just like the GPA, the MCAT may be thought of as a hurdle every pre-med must cross. And similar to the GPA, this bar sits at different heights for different schools and applicants. Graphs created from the most recent AAMC data are on the following pages.

Academics

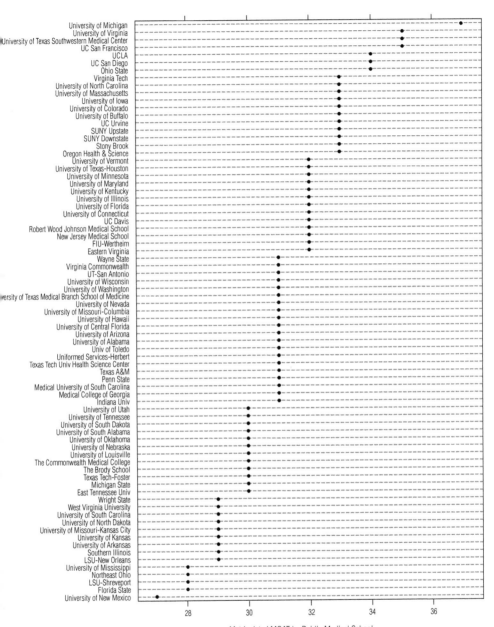

Matriculated MCAT by Public Medical School

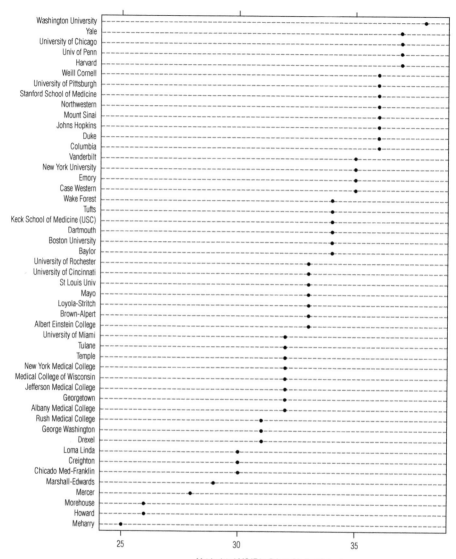

Matriculated MCAT by Private Medical School

Academics

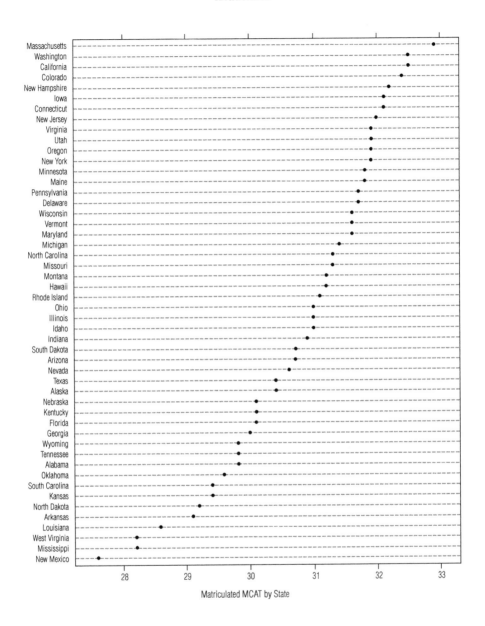

Matriculated MCAT by State

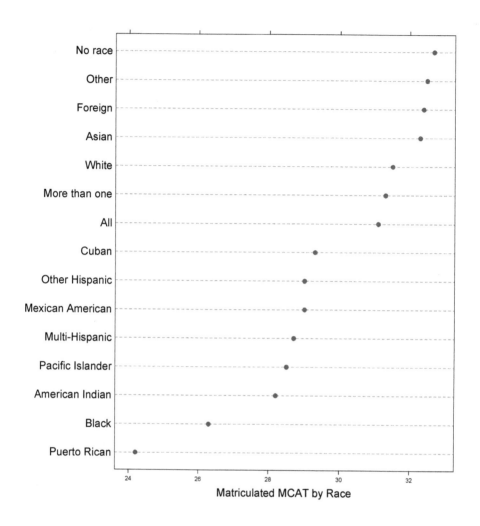

Matriculated MCAT by Race

Academics

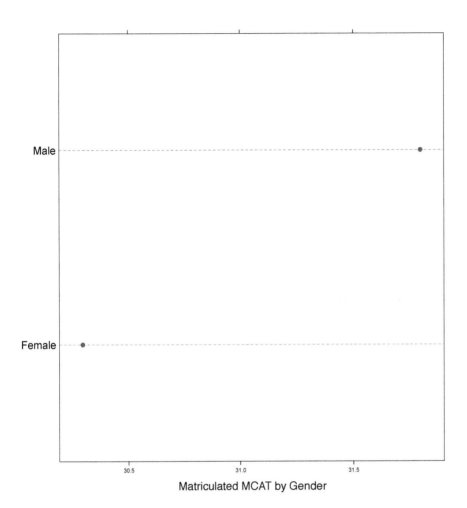

Matriculated MCAT by Gender

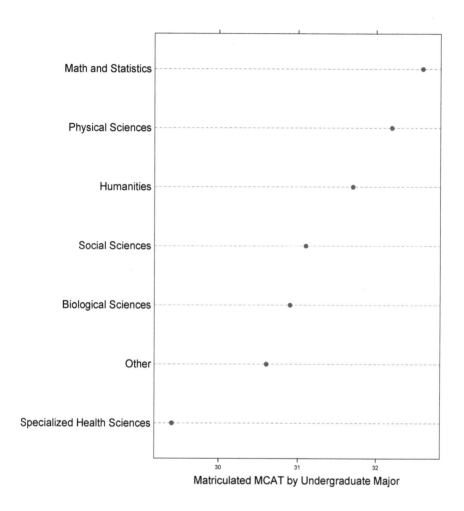

Matriculated MCAT by Undergraduate Major

As you can see from the data, scoring above a 30 bodes well for you getting into medical school. Interestingly, the MCAT average range is wider for private than public schools, with some of the less competitive private schools having MCAT averages well below 30. Be careful when looking at the public school graph. You may be enticed to apply to the University of New Mexico because it has the lowest average MCAT scores of all state schools. But unless you are lucky enough to be a New Mexico resident, your chances of getting in, even with a 45 MCAT, are slim. Remember, public schools give an overwhelming advantage to in-state residents.

When it comes to race, the AAMC MCAT data is similar to the GPA data with certain ethnic minorities having lower average scores. But different than the GPA, men have a significantly higher average MCAT score than women. Further, the MCAT data shows humanities majors scoring relatively higher on the MCAT when compared to social science, biological science, other, and specialized health science majors.

Rule of 65

Your head may be spinning with all of these graphs and talk of GPA and MCAT hurdles. To simplify how medical schools view GPA and MCAT scores, I will use a pulley metaphor. Think of the MCAT and GPA as separate strings of a pulley system. The higher the GPA, the lower the MCAT can be. The lower the GPA, the higher the MCAT needs to be. If you have amazing grades, you simply need to show those marks were not a fluke. If you have faltered in certain classes or are taking a non-traditional path to medical school, the MCAT is your chance to prove you have mastered the required basic science and language skills. Some admissions committees follow the "Rule of 65" which is as follows:

If GPA x 10 + MCAT > 65, then you have likely passed the academic bar required for medical school admissions.

For example, if you have a GPA of 3.7 and MCAT of 31, then:

3.7 x 10 + 31 = 68

Since 68 is greater than 65, the medical school admissions committee will likely move on to assess other parts of your application. Of course, this is not a strict rule and is certainly not followed by every medical school admissions committee. Take it simply as a guide to see how you are doing. And remember, every pre-med's academic achievement will be assessed differently by medical school admissions committees based on the characteristics discussed above.

MCAT Changes

The brand new MCAT, referred to as MCAT^{2015}, rolls out in 2015 and will affect pre-meds applying for entry to medical school in 2016 and later. The AAMC spent three years studying how to improve the MCAT to better reflect recent advances in medical science and the need for "softer" skills to excel as a physician. They have created a comprehensive, 153-page *Preview Guide for the MCAT^{2015}* available for free download at https://www.aamc.org/students/applying/mcat/. This document covers every detail of the MCAT change including sample questions.

Here's a summary of the changes to expect:

Biological sciences section is now called, "Biological and Biochemical Foundations of Living Systems."

Physical sciences section is now called, "Chemical and Physical Foundations of Biological Systems."

○ Both of these sections, referred to collectively as the "natural sciences" will continue to test concepts in biology, general and organic chemistry, biochemistry, and physics and will be updated to reflect the information medical school faculty believe is most important for success in medical school.

Addition of a new social and behavioral science section called, "Psychological, Social, and Biological Foundations of Behavior."

○ This section will test knowledge of introductory psychiatry and sociology, in addition to biological concepts relating to mental process and behavior. Understanding of basic research methods and statistics will also be tested.

Verbal reasoning section is now called, "Critical Analysis and Reasoning Skills."

○ This section requires analysis and application of information provided in passages from social science and humanities disciplines. Passages will include subjects such as ethics, philosophy, cross-cultural studies, and population health. Similar to the previous verbal reasoning section, you may be asked to decipher the tone and overall view of the passage author.

Just like the current physical sciences, verbal reasoning, and biological sciences sections, the MCAT[2015]'s four sections will be scored on a 1-15 scale. Four sections, four scores.

The expected breakdown of the test sections, questions, and time limits is as follows:

TEST SECTION	QUESTIONS	TIME
Biological and Biochemical Foundations of Living Systems	65	95 minutes
Chemical and Physical Foundations of Biological Systems	65	95 minutes
Psychological, Social, and Biological Foundations of Behavior	65	95 minutes
Critical Analysis and Reasoning Skills	60	90 minutes

The AAMC will continue to offer low-cost test preparation materials. Already on the AAMC MCAT[2015] website (https://www.aamc.org/students/applying/mcat/mcat2015/) you can find an informational video featuring advice on how to prepare for the new exam. In 2014, a full-length practice test will be posted on the site allowing pre-meds to simulate the actual test, and *The Official Guide to MCAT[2015]* will be released. Further, in 2015, AAMC will release a second full-length practice exam.

As with all new standardized exams, there will be considerable anxiety from both pre-meds and admissions committees regarding how to interpret the scores. While the AAMC works out the kinks, it is possible the MCAT will carry slightly less weight than usual. Though you may see this as a good thing, it will make your GPA only more important.

Whew, we have reached the end of the Academics Bucket. The pre-med academic requirements certainly aren't simple. But instead of feeling overwhelmed, use the information to take action. It is always easier to accomplish a task when you know what is required of you.

MYTH BUSTERS: ACADEMICS

The pre-med rumor mill has created the following myths. All of these myths have been busted.

- Pre-med is a major.
- You need to major in science to get into medical school.
- You have to go straight from college to medical school.
- If you don't have a 4.0 GPA, you can't get into medical school.
- A perfect MCAT score guarantees admission to medical school.

FILL IT UP

Use the area below to take notes on filling the Academics Bucket

....

....

....

....

....

....

....

....

....

....

....

....

....

CHAPTER 2

Research

Now that you have a thorough understanding of the pre-med academic requirements, let's move on to the second of the Six Buckets: Research.

Research Definition

Do you need to perform research to get into medical school? Yes. But "research" may not mean exactly what you think. Research does not have to involve pipetting in the lab or creating mutant rats. Laboratory research is an excellent way to delve deeper into basic science and work with other brilliant investigators trying to solve a problem, but it is not the only type of research available to pre-meds.

In the eyes of medical school admissions committees, research is defined as any activity that involves asking a question and then trying to answer it. You form a hypothesis and attempt to solve it.

The goal of your pre-med research experience is to prove to medical school admissions committees your talent for analytical thinking and problem solving.

Many activities fall under this broader definition of research. The following list of research activities shows the vastness of the research world, and these are only a few examples. Do not be limited by stereotypes or expectations. There is no need to join a lab just because all your friends say you need to work in basic science to get into medical school. The academic requirements of medicine almost all require basic science lab experience. After completing these academic prerequisites, you can retire the pipette if you desire. But, you do need to perform some sort of research. Use these lists to get the creative juices flowing.

BASIC SCIENCE/LABORATORY RESEARCH

» Study GAD65 antigen therapy in recently diagnosed type 1 diabetes mellitus

» Test novel use of TNF-alpha antagonist in Grave's disease treatment

» Investigate thrombolytic activity of different strains of β-hemolytic *Streptococcus* bacteria

» Analyze vector-borne diseases in avian species

» Design experiments to study protein shift during ultrafiltration/diafiltration process of hemodialysis

» Develop method for quantifying neurofilament regeneration through biomimetic 3D scaffolds

» Create *in vivo* models to study effect of novel cardiovascular treatments for pharmaceutical company

» Research whether chloride dioxide can serve as effective sterilization method

» Use mouse model to explore genomic instability's role in cancer development

» Examine effects of glucose levels on endogenous morphine production

CLINICAL/POPULATION-BASED RESEARCH

» Study HIV transmission rates from mother to child in Uganda

» Analyze health disparities of Costa Ricans versus Nicaraguans in San Pablo de Heredia, Costa Rica

» Perform language tests on elderly individuals with and without dementia to determine if subtle language deficits can predict development of Alzheimer's disease

» Study effects of regular exercise on breast cancer survival

» Attempt to alter nutrition-related behaviors of physicians through continuing education involving nutrition experts

» Use fMRI to study effect of smoking cessation on depression

» Improve supply chain to make pharmaceuticals more affordable for HIV patients in sub-Saharan Africa

» Investigate impact of new neuroleptic drug on intractable seizure population

» Explore alcohol counseling's impact on addicts admitted to rehabilitation unit

» Examine source of post-earthquake cholera outbreak in Haiti

HEALTH POLICY RESEARCH

» Evaluate how states fund immunizations for a congressionally-sponsored immunization finance study

» Draft white paper on global payment systems versus fee-for-service payments for health care consulting firm

» Analyze Medicare data to determine range of charges for appendicitis

» Study rate of health care errors in hospital system

» Create list of health care practices that do not offer value and should be de-funded

» Determine legal validity of health care mandate in US

» Investigate utilization of emergency departments versus primary care physicians in Medicaid patient cohort

» Explore policy changes to increase speed of generic pharmaceutical introduction to market

» Create questionnaire to study how physician practices would change with malpractice reform

» Research feasibility of telemedical specialist consults in rural community

BIOTECHNICAL RESEARCH

» Research most cost-effective way to implement electronic health record system at local clinic

» Use nanotechnology to develop handheld laboratory analyzers to be used at bedside

» Design mechanical straw mechanism that allows quadriplegic patients to control drinking from wheelchair-mounted water bottle

» Develop e-learning tool in game format to disseminate cancer research findings

» Create online program allowing clinics to track needs of chronically ill patients

» Build solar-powered generator to run medical equipment when primary source of electricity fails in resource-poor settings

» Study impact of cell phone application technology in patients trying to lose weight

» Construct sustainable water filtration system for village in Peru

» Employ gaming system to teach pediatric cancer patients importance of taking medications

» Invent computer program that assists disaster relief organizations with communications during search and rescue efforts

HUMANITIES RESEARCH

» Study economic impact of microfinance on women's club in Afghanistan

» Write thesis on history of surgical techniques from time of Hippocrates to present

» Chronicle dying language from indigenous population in Andes Mountains

» Compose book on history of international pharmaceutical policies

» Investigate scientists to be included in *Most Notable American Woman* series

» Analyze socioeconomic causes contributing to Sudanese civil war

» Chart movements of pandas in China to study effect of climate change

» Create documentary on role of Southern Lebanese Army in Israeli-Palestinian conflict

» Assist economics professor in research on causes of 2008 financial collapse

» Evaluate use of art as means of women's expression in Burma

Are you inspired? I hope the point is now clear – "research" has an extremely broad meaning. Sure, the laboratory is an excellent place to gain research experience, but it is not the only place. The key is to find a problem you are interested in solving or a question you'd like to answer, and then look for a solution.

How to Find a Research Position

When attempting to find a research position, focus first on what subjects fascinate you and what problems you would like to solve. Then try to find long-term opportunities allowing room for advancement and independent projects. There is no need to do a different research project every year of college. In fact, medical school admissions committees prefer you stay with one experience for a longer period of time than hop around each semester or year from one research opportunity to another. Remember, getting into medical school is not about checking the boxes. It's about doing what you love, doing it well, and being able to use the experience to show the admissions committees you have the characteristics and skills required to be an excellent physician.

Do you need to publish a research paper to get into medical school? No. But it certainly doesn't hurt. Being named an author in a research publication, abstract, or presentation provides evidence that you have played an integral role in the research team. But getting published is certainly not a requirement of being pre-med. If you don't have a publication opportunity, attending academic research conferences is another way you can show commitment to research. Conferences are often expensive but offer steep discounts for students. Or perhaps your research team could sponsor you and pay part of the conference fee.

Some pre-meds find obtaining the "right" research opportunity difficult. Discovering a research experience that fits your interests and goals will certainly take time. But with persistence, I guarantee you can find an interesting research opportunity. Try not to jump into the first project that presents itself unless it feels right. You hope to be in this research position for years, so don't take the decision lightly. Find a research venue where you feel comfortable with your colleagues, enjoy the subject, learn new skills, and make a contribution.

Pre-meds often do not know where to start looking for research experiences. It certainly can be a daunting task. Begin by determining what kind of research you would like to do. For example, would you like to assist with basic science, clinical, health policy, biotechnical, or humanities research? Or is there a completely different type of research you want to pursue? Once you have made this decision, narrow your focus to a particular part of this general research area. For example, do you want to study genetic markers of chronic disease in flies, cardiac disease in neonates, insurance premiums for patients with pre-existing conditions, implantable biomedical devices, or economic policies of communist countries?

Now that you have narrowed your interests, it's time to turn to your network. Do your family, friends, or colleagues know of anyone doing research in this area? Do your professors have any research leads? How about your family doctor? Does he or she have any research connections? Does your university's office of career services or pre-med group have online databases of professors looking for research assistants? When searching for a new opportunity, having a personal introduction is often very helpful. Use your network and see if anyone can guide you to a research experience.

In addition to using your personal network to find a research opportunity, you can also hit the Internet. It is usually best to start with the website of your own university or a local academic institution, and then expand your search from there. Go to your university's website and search for professors performing research in your area of interest. In this Internet age, most professors keep their resumes online.

I know specifics can be helpful, so let me provide an example. Let us say you just read an article in the newspaper about how iPhone applications are being used to help diabetic patients lose weight and you are interested in working on research investigating how mobile technology can help chronically ill patients. You go to your university's website and search for "mobile technology and diabetes research." From the results, you find the school of public health has partnered with the endocrinology department on a trial studying how a smart phone application can assist diabetics with eating low-sugar foods. Dr. Bernard is listed as the principal investigator.

Now it is time to contact Dr. Bernard. When making this first contact, introduce yourself and then be specific about the commitment you can make. For example, you may be able to offer five hours per week of volunteer time to help with the investigation. Or you could be looking for a full-time paid position for the next year. In this initial contact, clearly layout how much time you can spend on the research and whether you are looking for a volunteer or paid position. Of course, being able to volunteer your time on a consistent basis will make you more desirable than if you need to be paid. Also, in this first contact it is important to emphasize the characteristics and skills you bring to the job. Even if you have not performed research before, you certainly have developed useful qualities, such as being self-motivated, well-organized, and team-oriented, likely to help in any setting. Finally, you should include an updated resume in this initial contact.

Here is an example of a research query e-mail:

Dear Dr. Bernard,

I am a sophomore pre-med at Maryland State University majoring in computer science and am interested in the use of mobile applications to improve the health of chronically ill patients. While performing research on the Internet, I came upon your project studying the impact of a smart phone application on the diet of diabetics. I would love to get involved in this project and can volunteer my time as a research assistant for 10 hours per week during the semester and 40 hours per week during the summer.

I believe my computer savvy, organizational abilities, and communication skills will serve your project well. My academic background in computer science has made me well versed in both computer programming and database management. I am also interested in gaining more experience with statistical programming and have been teaching myself SAS. In addition, I have learned to juggle multiple extracurricular and academic commitments, having worked 20-hours per week while volunteering 10 hours per week in the hospital last semester, and am confident the organization skills I have honed will help me excel as your research assistant. Further, I feel comfortable communicating with people from all backgrounds, a skill I developed while working as a university tour guide, waitress, and basketball coach.

I am able to start at the beginning of the semester. My resume is attached for your reference. I look forward to hearing from you and am happy to stop by your office to discuss this further.

Sincerely,
Jane Dositrite

As you can see in this example e-mail, Jane hits the most important elements of an initial research query:

1. Brief introduction with statement of interest
2. Time commitment and type of position desired (volunteer vs. paid)
3. Succinct discussion of skills/qualities/characteristics that will make you an asset to the project (often best to include three as humans think best in groups of three)
4. Conclusion with reference to resume and willingness to speak in person

As with many things in life, research queries are likely to result in more rejections than acceptances. It is important to have a thick skin and not take the rejections personally. If a professor does not have a position available, you can always ask if he or she knows of any other professors or principal investigators looking for research assistants. In general, you will have to send out at least ten research queries to obtain a position. But with hard work, you are very likely to find a positive experience.

In addition to using your network and the Internet to find research opportunities, there are also specific research internships and fellowships offered to pre-med students. These opportunities usually run during the summer months and are at times highly competitive. See below for a list of some of the best pre-med research websites and the most prestigious research fellowships:

BEST PRE-MED RESEARCH WEBSITES

AAMC

https://www.aamc.org/members/great/61052/great_summerlinks.html

The AAMC has collated summer undergraduate research programs by medical school sponsor. This should be your first stop for summer research opportunities.

Rochester Institute of Technology (RIT)

http://people.rit.edu/gtfsbi/Symp/summer.htm

Tom Frederick of Rochester Institute of Technology maintains an impressive website listing summer research internships in the life sciences and breaks each opportunity into categories such as, "Opportunities in Biomedical Research and for Pre-Medical Studies Students," "Opportunities for Minority and Underrepresented Students," and "Opportunities that may consider First-Year Undergraduates." Mr. Frederick focuses on paid opportunities but does include volunteer options.

Columbia

http://www.columbia.edu/cu/biology/ug/intern.html

Columbia has created a website that lists research opportunities in New York City and beyond including sections on biomedical laboratory research, ecology and environmental studies, and marine biology, among others.

MOST PRESTIGIOUS RESEARCH FELLOWSHIPS

National Science Foundation (NSF)

http://www.nsf.gov/crssprgm/reu/index.jsp

The NSF funds undergraduate research experiences through its Research Experience for Undergraduates (REU) Sites program. A REU Site is comprised of about ten undergraduate students who work in the host institutions' research programs. Students are associated with a specific project and receive stipends for their work. Each individual REU site runs its own application process. Only US citizens and permanent residents are eligible.

National Institutes of Health (NIH)

https://www.training.nih.gov/programs

The NIH offers many research fellowships. One of the most popular is the Summer Internship Program in Biomedical Research (SIP) (**https://www.training.nih.gov/programs/sip**). This program provides funding for undergraduates to spend the summer working intimately with some of the greatest scientists in the country. In 2012, the NIH started the Community College Summer Enrichment Program (CCSEP) (**https://www.training.nih.gov/ccsep_home_page**) that aims to bring more community college students into the SIP. If you have already graduated from college and are interested in spending a year or two doing research, you can apply to the Postbaccalaureate Intramural Research Training Award (**https://www.training.nih.gov/programs/postbac_irta**).

Howard Hughes Medical Institute (HHMI) http://www.hhmi.org
HHMI is a nonprofit medical research institute founded in 1953 by Howard Hughes and located in Chevy Chase, Maryland. Its goal is to advance biomedical research and science education in the US. HHMI has a searchable database on its website (**http://www.hhmi.org/grants/search/scienceopp/index.php?view=s4squeryform**) allowing you to input "college undergraduates," location, and text search fields. When I searched the database for "college undergraduates" and "any location," the database showed over 50 possible research opportunities at universities all over the country. Be sure to check back often, as the database is updated regularly when new opportunities arise.

HOW TO OBTAIN A RESEARCH POSITION

Determine broad area of research interest (basic science, clinical, health policy, biotechnical, humanities research, other)

↓

Narrow focus to a particular research area

↓   ↓   ↓

Contact Network   Search Internet   Research Fellowships

↓   ↓   ↓

Send query e-mail/resume   Send query e-mail/resume   Apply

↓

Follow-up e-mail/application responses

Many clients have complained about negative research experiences, but express concern that leaving a research project after one semester will look bad on their medical school applications. It is certainly true admissions committees prefer to see commitment in pre-med activities, but it is not worth tolerating a negative experience in order to have something look good on your application. If you are miserable, then make a cordial break with the laboratory or research team and find another opportunity. Remember, if you do what you love, you will do it well, and it will look good on your application.

MYTH BUSTERS: RESEARCH
The pre-med rumor mill has created the following myths. All of these myths have been busted.

- You can get into medical school without research experience.
- You have to do laboratory research to gain admission to medical school.
- The research you did as a history major does not count as research.
- You have to be published to get into medical school.
- All research positions are paid.
- It is impossible to obtain a research position if you do not have a direct connection to a researcher.

FILL IT UP

Use the area below to take notes on filling the Research Bucket

Community Service

S ervice lies at the core of medicine. Whether working as an internist or pathologist, you will spend every day trying to improve the lives of others. Because service is such an integral part of being a physician, medical school admissions committees want to see you excel at helping others. Thus, Community Service is the third of the Six Buckets.

Similar to research, community service has a broad definition and refers to any activity where you are helping someone else. You can be creative when deciding how to serve the community and need not limit volunteer experiences to the medical setting. You just need to help other people.

Admissions committees strongly prefer you show consistency and leadership in community service activities. For example, it is more impressive to volunteer in the emergency department for four years and receive promotions from volunteer intern to volunteer trainer to volunteer supervisor than to participate in a one-week community health fair for underserved populations each year in college. I refer to short-term community service experiences as "one-offs." Spending a day coaching a basketball camp, helping run a blood drive, or washing cars for charity are all one-offs. These one-off activities may be wonderful and should be pursued if you enjoy them. But spending one day helping others does not have enough substance to be included in your medical school application. When choosing your community service activities, think commitment and leadership. To spur your creative spirit, I have created a list of example community service experiences.

Feed

- Provide healthy meals every Sunday night to a disadvantaged community with Sunday Suppers
- Serve at soup kitchen connected to women's shelter
- Collect donations for local food bank
- Deliver food to ill and elderly citizens with Meals on Wheels
- Start affordable health food store in impoverished inner-city neighborhood

Clothe

- Gather suit donations for homeless individuals to wear on job interviews
- Create inexpensive flip-flops for children living in Amazon Basin to prevent soil-transmitted parasites
- Design culturally-appropriate clothing for impoverished community in Burma using donated t-shirts
- Run bake sale to raise money for flood relief in Pakistan
- Knit booties and blankets for premature infants

Build/Design

- Build wells in Zimbabwe village with no clean water source
- Construct homes with Habitat for Humanity
- Design power-free stove to be used safely indoors
- Devise simple IT solution to show Peruvian farmers how to best plant fields
- Invent solar-based generator to be used when electricity fails in Rwanda

Educate

- Teach science to at-risk, inner-city youth
- Tutor child with Down's syndrome
- Show nursing home residents how to create video diaries of their lives
- Provide sex education to adolescents in Kenyan ghetto
- Serve as English teacher in Siberia

Entertain

- Teach Mahjong to nursing home residents and then organize tournaments
- Volunteer for Clowns Without Borders
- Play guitar at children's hospital
- Organize play to benefit Oxfam
- Establish dance program for injured soldiers

Improve Health

- Drive elderly patient to chemotherapy treatments
- Hold babies orphaned by Tsunami in Indonesia
- Volunteer in emergency department or local free clinic
- Start art therapy course for troubled youth in Brazil
- Wash feet of homeless at free clinic

Finding a community service project tends to be easier than obtaining a research experience. Opportunities to donate your time are all around you. Check your college clubs, local religious organizations, and, of course, the Internet. So many people are searching for meaningful ways to help that websites have popped up to organize the plethora of service options in the US and around the world.

To assist with your community service search and provide a sense of the virtually limitless volunteer opportunities available, I have created an annotated list of general community service, international community service, and well-respected community and medical service organizations. I have also included a list of "gap year" organizations that assist in finding overseas placements for college graduates who want to take time off prior to entering graduate school. As mentioned in the Academics Bucket, no rule exists stating you must go directly from college to medical school. In fact, maturity and experience gained in a gap year or years often improve your chances of medical school admissions.

The list of general community service organizations provides websites with searchable databases of volunteer opportunities. Many US states, counties, and cities have their own volunteer websites. I suggest typing "volunteer" and your geographic area of interest (*i.e.* "Volunteer Washington DC") into an Internet search engine in addition to surfing the sites below. I do not personally recommend any of these organizations or websites but offer them as a starting point for your search.

General Community Service Websites

Volunteer Solutions
http://volunteer.truist.com/

Volunteer Solutions has created a "Volunteer Matching Application" helping volunteer centers connect individuals to community service opportunities. The organization connects volunteers, nonprofit agencies, corporations, event organizers, and volunteer centers. You can search for volunteer opportunities based on interests, skills, and geographic location or by entering a keyword. You may also register to receive automatic emails that list volunteer opportunities matching your specific profile.

VolunteerMatch
http://www.volunteermatch.org/

VolunteerMatch aims to strengthen communities by making it easier for "good people and good causes" to connect. The website offers a searchable database to find volunteer opportunities or recruit volunteers based on location and keywords. More than 85,000 nonprofit organizations are registered.

United We Serve
http://www.serve.gov/

United We Serve is a nationwide service initiated by President Obama to help meet growing social needs resulting from the economic downturn. The initiative hopes to expand the impact of existing organizations by engaging new volunteers and encouraging volunteers to develop their own projects. Serve.gov allows you to create your own project, find a volunteer opportunity, and register your project to recruit volunteers.

Many pre-meds want to volunteer abroad. Here are a few well-established websites that offer international volunteer opportunity information.

International Community Service Websites

Global Volunteer Network
http://www.globalvolunteernetwork.org/3/

Started in 2001, Global Volunteer Network has sent over 15,000 volunteers abroad and offers 63 projects in 20 countries. This is a service you will have to pay for as they charge for the placement.

Volunteers For Peace
http://www.vfp.org

Founded in 1982, Volunteers For Peace promotes international
volunteerism as an "effective means of intercultural education,
service learning, and community development." The organization
offers over 3,000 projects in more than 100 countries. Projects
include volunteering with children, teaching English, restoring the
environment, and assisting with HIV/AIDS awareness projects. In
addition to international projects, Volunteers For Peace organizes
40-60 projects in the US. The registration fee is $350 regardless
of program length and covers food, accommodation, and work
materials for the project. This fee does not include travel costs.

International Volunteer Programs Association (IVPA)
http://www.volunteerinternational.org/

Given the tremendous interest in volunteering abroad but lack of
universal standards for volunteer organizations, the IVPA recognized
a need for an accrediting organization to provide unbiased
information about community service organizations. The IVPA
started an application process in 2007 to screen non-governmental
organizations involved in international volunteer work and
internship exchanges. It does not run its own volunteer programs.
Take a look at the organizations IVPA has accredited as they have
passed certain hurdles and are more likely to be on the up and up.

There are many community service organizations discussed frequently in the media, but perhaps you are unclear about what they
do and how to get involved. Here is an alphabetical list of groups
considered the giants of service. All of these organizations are well
respected and have organized volunteer programs.

Well-Respected Service Organizations

American Red Cross
http://www.redcross.org/en/volunteer

The American Red Cross aims to "provide compassionate care to those in need" and focuses on five main areas – disaster relief, supporting military families, blood donations, health and safety services, and international services. More than 90% of the organization's labor force are volunteers and the website lays out many ways to get involved.

Amnesty International
http://www.amnesty.org/

Amnesty International campaigns to end human rights abuses with its "global movement of more than three million supporters, members, and activists." Information on the US branch can be found at http://www.amnestyusa.org/. The organization offers ample volunteer opportunities (http://www.amnestyusa.org/get-involved/volunteer-positions-and-resources) in areas such as letter-writing campaigns, phone banking, and lobbying.

Big Brothers Big Sisters
http://www.bbbs.org

Big Brothers Big Sisters started when a New York City court clerk noticed more boys than usual coming through the courtroom and sought to find volunteer adults who could help many of these children stay out of trouble. Around the same time, the Ladies of Charity performed a similar role for girls who came through the courts and later became the Catholic Big Sisters. Big Brothers and Catholic Big Sisters merged in 1977 to become Big Brothers Big Sisters of America and continue to match volunteer mentors one-on-one with a child. To find a mentoring position in your area, visit http://www.bbbs.org/site/c.9iILl3NGKhK6F/b.5962345/k.E123/Volunteer_to_start_something.htm.

BRAC
http://www.brac.net/

BRAC is now the world's largest development organization. Started in Bangladesh in 1972, BRAC is "dedicated to alleviating poverty by empowering the poor to bring about change in their own lives." The organization helps a community struggling with poverty take control by using its own human and material resources. Now in 11 countries, BRAC offers both internship and volunteer opportunities that can be found at http://www.brac.net/content/get-involved-volunteers-interns#.UFyzSxhc4_o.

CARE International

http://www.care-international.org/

CARE describes itself as "a global confederation of 14 member organizations working together to end poverty." CARE works in over 80 countries supporting over 1,000 projects dedicated to fighting poverty. Most of the ways to get involved in CARE involve starting a student group, fundraising, or political advocacy. More details can be found at **http://www.care.org/getinvolved/index.asp**, including a helpful Student Action Kit.

Catholic Charities

http://www.catholiccharitiesusa.org/

Catholic Charities is one of the largest religious-based charitable organizations. The organization "works with individuals, families, and communities to help them meet their needs, address their issues, eliminate oppression, and build a just and compassionate society." Many volunteer opportunities exist in the organization, but you have to contact a local office. For example, the volunteer options in Washington, DC can be found at **http://www. catholiccharitiesdc.org/GetInvolved**. It is very common for service-oriented organizations to have a religious connection. If you want to work with an organization with a specific religious leaning, a quick Internet search will reveal many choices. Here are some of the many examples: American Baptist Foundation (**http://www. americanbaptistfdn.org/**), Lutheran Volunteer Corps (**www. lutheranvolunteercorps.org/**), Jewish Charities of America (**http:// www.jewishcoa.org/**), Islamic Relief (**http://www.irusa.org/**), Hindu Charities of America (**http://www.hinducharitiesforamerica.org/**), and Tzu Chi (**http://www.us.tzuchi.org/us/en/**).

City Year

http://www.cityyear.org

City Year's motto is, "Give a year. Change the world." Under the AmeriCorps (**www.americorps.gov/**) umbrella, City Year works to address the one million students who drop out of high school each year in the US. Half of these one million dropouts come from just 12% of schools. City Year is looking for "team players" who have leadership skills and are able to commit to ten months of full-time service dedicated to "providing academic support, attendance and positive behavior encouragement, and community and school improvements to disadvantaged communities." Applicants to City Year must have attended some college, be between the ages of 17 and 24, be a US citizen or permanent resident, have serviced no more than three terms in another Americorps program, and agree to a background check.

Girl Scouts/Boy Scouts

http://www.girlscouts.org/

More than just selling delicious cookies, the Girl Scouts aim to "build girls of courage, confidence, and character, who make the world a better place." There are ample volunteer opportunities, even if you were never a Girl Scout: **http://www.girlscouts.org/for_adults/ volunteering/**.

Boy Scouts
http://www.scouting.org/

The Boy Scouts provide "a program for young people that builds character, trains them in the responsibilities of participating citizenship, and develops personal fitness." Nearly 1.2 million adults volunteer to provide mentoring to Boy Scouts programs. For Boy Scouts volunteer opportunities, contact a local chapter in your area.

Habitat for Humanity
http://www.habitat.org/

Habitat for Humanity in a non-profit organization that has helped build over 500,000 affordable houses worldwide. Its goal is a world "where everyone has a decent place to live." Started in 1976 by Millard and Linda Fuller, the organization has ecumenical Christian roots but neither housing recipients nor volunteers are selected based on religion. The Habitat for Humanity model is centered on volunteer labor and donations with homes being sold to families at no profit and financed with affordable loans. The mortgage payments then fund more Habitat houses. Ready to roll up your sleeves and help build a house? Then visit **http://www.habitat.org/local/** to find your local Habitat affiliate and specific volunteer options.

International Federation of Red Cross and Red Crescent Societies (IFRC)
http://www.ifrc.org

IFRC is the international parent organization of national Red Cross and Red Crescent Societies, such as the American Red Cross (see above). It advertises itself as the world's largest humanitarian network reaching greater than 150 million people through the work of over 13 million volunteers. The website points potential volunteers to the local Red Cross or Red Crescent Society in your home nation. If you want to volunteer with IFRC abroad, start local and ask to go global through one of the partner national societies.

International Rescue Committee (IRC)
http://www.rescue.org/volunteering

The International Rescue Committee, founded in 1933 at the request of Albert Einstein, focuses on helping refugees forced to flee from war or disaster. In an emergency, the IRC arrives on the scene within 72 hours to offer refugees life-saving assistance. In the US, the IRC helps refugees thrive in their new country. Most IRC volunteer opportunities are located in the US and involve mentoring and teaching refugees and administrative duties, but occasional international volunteer opportunities are posted. The volunteer application includes a written application, orientation, interview, and background check.

Kiva
http://www.kiva.org/

Kiva is one of the leading microfinance non-profit organizations and aims to "connect people through lending to alleviate poverty." Most of Kiva's volunteer opportunities come in the form of internships in the San Francisco office. However, the Kiva Fellows Program involves living in a host country of the partner microfinance institutions for a minimum of 12 weeks. In addition, there are interesting opportunities to volunteer as a loan editor or translator. See **http://www.kiva.org/volunteer.**

Meals on Wheels Association of America (MOWAA)
http://www.mowaa.org/

Meals on Wheels Association of America is composed of 5,000 local, community-based senior nutrition programs providing over one million meals to seniors in need each day. Some programs deliver meals directly to homes of seniors with limited mobility while others provide meals in locations like senior centers. MOWAA boasts an "army" of volunteers numbering between 800,000 and 1.7 million individuals who help deliver and prepare meals. To find a local program and volunteer visit **http://www.mowaa.org/Page.aspx?pid=396.**

National Park Service

http://www.nps.gov/getinvolved/volunteer.htm

The National Park Service is a government agency responsible for running the nearly 400 US national parks. The website provides a volunteer database searchable by park name, state, or zip code. Volunteers perform jobs as varied as working the visitor center desk, guiding nature walks, and designing park websites. The volunteer brochure provides a helpful map detailing the location of every national park.

Oxfam

http://www.oxfam.org/

Oxfam states its mission as, "We believe we can end poverty and injustice, as part of a global movement for change." Networking together 17 organizations in greater than 90 countries, Oxfam works directly with communities to help individuals suffering from poverty improve their lives and have a voice in decisions that affect them. The organization focuses on development, emergency response, campaigning, advocacy, and policy research. Oxfam heavily relies on volunteers and you can find available opportunities at http://www.oxfam.org/en/getinvolved/volunteer.

Peace Corps
http://www.peacecorps.gov/

The Peace Corps, a US federal government agency dedicated to world peace and friendship, started after Senator John F. Kennedy challenged students at the University of Michigan in 1960 to serve their country in the cause of peace by living and working in developing countries. Since that time, over 200,000 Peace Corps Volunteers have served in 139 host countries to work on issues including education, youth and community development, health, technology, agriculture, and environment. The total time commitment is 27 months. Volunteers are not paid a salary during this time, but receive small stipends for transition funds, travel to and from the country of service, living and housing expenses, and medical/dental insurance. There is no placement fee.

Save the Children
http://www.savethechildren.org

Save the Children is dedicated to, not surprisingly, helping kids in the US and around the world. The organization responds to disaster and civil conflicts and works to resolve the issues of poverty, hunger, illiteracy, and disease that affect children daily. Save the Children has many volunteer opportunities in both the US (Washington, DC and Westport, CT) and abroad. Check out **http://www.savethechildren.org/site/c.8rKLIXMGIpI4E/b.6540957/k.7CF9/Volunteer_Opportunities.htm** for details.

Teach for America
http://www.teachforamerica.org/

Teach for America looks to provide impoverished children living in the US with better educational opportunities by hiring a diverse group of individuals who will teach for two years in a low-income community. Application requirements include a bachelor's degree by the time of summer training, 2.5 minimum GPA, and US citizen or permanent resident status. The application process involves a written application and interview. Teach for America salaries range from $25,500 to $51,000 depending on location and cost of living. All teachers also receive health and retirement benefits.

United Nations
www.unv.org

The United Nations has a branch that contributes to peace and development through volunteerism worldwide. The headquarters is situated in Bonn, Germany, but the program is active in 130 countries and mobilizes over 7,700 volunteers each year. The online volunteering service (**http://www.onlinevolunteering.org/en/index. html**) offers a database to connect development organizations directly with online volunteers who can provide services and advice over the Internet.

United Way
http://www.unitedway.org/take-action/volunteer/

The United Way traces its roots back to 1887, when a Denver woman, a priest, two ministers, and a rabbi recognized the need for cooperative action to address the city's welfare problems. They created an organization that collected funds for local charities and coordinated relief services, referred clients to cooperating agencies, and made emergency assistance grants. Today, the United Way focuses on creating a world, "where all individuals and families achieve their human potential through education, income stability, and healthy lives." The volunteer page has a location-specific database for education and health volunteer opportunities.

Given you are pre-med, it is likely you have an interest in joining one of the many health-related service organizations. Remember, all of your community service does not have to directly relate to doctoring, but volunteering with a health-related group certainly does not hurt. Unfortunately, prior to obtaining your medical education and licensing, it can be somewhat difficult to do more than market and fundraise for many of these well-respected health service non-profits. But who knows? Perhaps a college fundraising campaign for Doctors Without Borders could lead you to a year-long medical mission once you become a physician.

Well-Respected Medical Service Organizations

Doctors Without Borders/Medecins Sans Frontieres (MSF)
http://www.msf.org/

Referred to as "MSF" by most of the world, Doctors Without Borders is one of the most respected international humanitarian organizations delivering emergency aid to people affected by natural disasters, armed conflict, epidemics, and exclusion from healthcare. They are known to work in areas of dire need where few other organizations will go. To join MSF in a medical capacity requires a medical or nursing degree and the minimum commitment generally runs nine months. For more information on US information sessions and opportunities visit **http://www.doctorswithoutborders.org/**.

Health Volunteers Overseas (HVO)
http://www.hvousa.org/

Health Volunteers Overseas focuses on sending trained medical personnel to international locations in order to educate local medical staff. The group currently supports 85 projects in more than 25 countries and focuses on teaching anesthesia, dermatology, hand surgery, hematology, internal medicine, nursing education, oral health, orthopedics, oncology, pediatrics, physical therapy, and wound care. Most placements are for one month. A helpful "frequently asked questions" page provides information explaining how HVO differs from other direct care organizations like MSF, International Medical Corps, and Merlin: **http://www.hvousa.org/ volunteerToolkit/faqs.shtml**.

International Medical Corps (IMC)

http://internationalmedicalcorps.org/

Founded in 1984, the International Medical Corps focuses on saving lives through health care training, in addition to relief and development programs. You will find members of this organization alongside MSF volunteers in disaster and humanitarian emergencies, but they often stay long after other groups have left, focusing on educating local providers on long-term care. Like MSF, most volunteer opportunities are open to trained professionals; however, IMC does offer administrative and programmatic volunteer opportunities in the US and a competitive Graduate Internship Program. See **http:// careers.internationalmedicalcorps.org/Volunteer.html**.

Mercy Ships

http://www.mercyships.org/

Since 1978, Mercy Ships has operated hospital ships to provide healthcare to developing nations. As with most health care–related organizations, Mercy Ships is generally looking for skilled health care workers as you can see on their volunteer page **http://www. mercyships.org/opportunities/**. However, they do have "Mercy Teams," an opportunity for non-medical personnel to volunteer on a shorter-term basis.

Merlin

http://www.merlin.org.uk/

Merlin is a British health charity that sends medical experts to sites of international emergencies, such as areas afflicted by natural disasters or armed conflicts. It does not send volunteers overseas, but has opportunities to get involved through paid work. See **http:// www.merlin.org.uk/jobs**.

Partners in Health
http://www.pih.org/

Founded by Harvard doctor Paul Farmer and President of the World
Bank Jim Kim and made famous by Tracey Kidder's book *Mountains
Beyond Mountains*, Partners in Health "uses all of the means at our
disposal" to make people well when they fall ill, "from pressuring
drug manufacturers, to lobbying policy makers, to providing medical
care and social services." The organization mainly works in Peru,
Siberia, and Haiti, and it relies more on low-paid workers than on
volunteers. Employment opportunities are available at **http://www.
pih.org/pages/employment/openings/**.

VSO International
http://www.vsointernational.org/

VSO is an international organization using volunteers to help
overcome poverty. The organization works in many areas of
development, including health. Given that VSO is based around
a volunteer work force, it has many service opportunities for
skilled medical personnel. Like most international organizations,
the volunteer positions are arranged by local VSO websites. For
example, here are the volunteer openings from the United Kingdom
(UK) website: **http://www.vso.org.uk/volunteer/opportunities/
health/index.asp**.

In British parlance, a "gap year" refers to taking time off in
between studies. This can be between high school and college or
college and graduate school. Many organizations and companies
have popped up in the UK and beyond to provide gap year students with opportunities to travel, learn, and volunteer abroad. Not
surprisingly, most charge a placement fee in addition to the costs

of travel, accommodation, and food. Here are some of the leading gap-year focused organizations:

GAP YEAR OPPORTUNITIES	
Raleigh International	http://www.raleighinternational.org/
World Challenge Expeditions	http://www.world-challenge.co.uk/
Project Trust	http://www.projecttrust.org.uk/
Latitude Global Volunteering	http://www.lattitude.org.uk/
BSES Expeditions	http://www.bses.org.uk/
Greenforce	http://www.greenforce.org/
Challenges Worldwide	http://challengesworldwide.org/
African Conservation Experience	http://www.conservationafrica.net/

Isn't it amazing how many organizations are trying to help the world? The opportunities to get involved are astounding. But as with searching for any opportunity, it is important to do your homework before accepting a volunteer position. Here are some questions to consider when finding a community service experience:

- Does the organization have a good reputation?
- What is the organization's mission and does it align with your values?
- Is it politically or religiously-affiliated, and is this important to you?
- How is it funded?
- Is it well organized?

▸ Can you make a genuine positive contribution to the organization?

▸ What are volunteers' responsibilities?

▸ Who supervises the volunteers?

▸ What is the minimum and maximum time commitment?

▸ Do possibilities for advancement/more responsibility exist?

▸ Does the organization charge volunteer fees? If so, what do the fees cover?

▸ Does volunteering with this organization put you in danger? How is safety addressed?

▸ What are the application requirements?

▸ Have your friends or family members volunteered with this group before?

▸ Can the organization put you in contact with previous volunteers?

Since volunteer and development organizations live off of donations, many evaluation lists have emerged to help donors make informed decisions. Appraisals of community service organizations, such as the *Global Journals'* "Top 100 NGOs" (http://theglobaljournal.net/top100NGOs/) may help you determine the quality of a group you are interested in joining.

Many volunteer opportunities require application or placement fees. These fees can sometimes reach into the thousands. It is most common for international organizations to request a fee as they claim to spend considerable resources ensuring volunteers have safe and fulfilling trips. I personally find it difficult to pay in order to volunteer my time, but some fees seem reasonable. Before you sign on to a volunteer experience, be sure you know the exact charges.

Safety in community service is rarely discussed but should be at the forefront of your decision-making when it comes to volunteering, particularly when traveling abroad. I made this mistake when offered a chance to travel to Haiti days after the 2010 earthquake. Because I was so excited by the opportunity, I did not perform a full review of the organization's safety plan. Though I returned in one piece, the volunteer group certainly experienced some harrowing moments that could have been avoided if a proper safety plan had been initiated prior to travel. Research the safety record of the organization you are about to join. How is safety specifically addressed by the organization? Who is responsible for your well-being? Does anyone speak the native language? Is evacuation insurance offered or do you have to purchase it yourself? Bottom line – be safe.

MYTH BUSTERS: COMMUNITY SERVICE
The pre-med rumor mill has created the following myths. All of these myths have been busted.

- All community service needs to be medically related to count for medical school admissions.
- It is better to obtain multiple "one-off" community service experiences than to stay with one organization for a longer period.
- Medical schools only want pre-meds to volunteer in the US.
- Pre-meds can't do any medically related volunteer work because they have no hard skills.
- Volunteer organizations never charge a fee.
- Safety is not an issue worth worrying about when doing community service.

FILL IT UP

Use the area below to take notes on filling
the Community Service Bucket

CHAPTER 4

Extracurriculars

The word "extracurricular," by strict definition, refers to any activity outside of the classroom. But in the context of medical school admissions, I use extracurricular to mean any experience that does not fit into the Academics, Research, Community Service, or Clinical Experience Buckets.

Extracurricular activities are a great way to stand out in the medical school admissions process. This is another chance to be creative and follow your passions. Admissions committee members may not remember you had a 3.7 GPA, but they will likely remember you climbed 50 14,000-foot mountains in Colorado over the last 5 years, or speak fluent Gaelic, or collect classic bicycles and auction them off for charity, or have worked for five years in Silicon Valley. Do not be afraid to follow your passions, even if they do not directly relate to medicine. Your extracurricular experiences will contribute not only to your medical school admissions chances, but will help you live a happy, well-balanced life. These activities often continue through medical school and beyond and make you who you are. When choosing extracurricular activities, the same rule applies to them as to every other pre-med experience: focus on commitment and leadership. Fewer stellar experiences are more powerful than many one-offs.

I am amazed how little thought many pre-meds put into extracurricular activities. A common misperception suggests these non-research, non-community service, non-clinical experiences are a waste of time. Nothing could be further from the truth. I have found extracurriculars often provide the defining experiences of life. How you spend your free time is a significant reflection of who you are as a person.

I have provided extracurricular examples on the following pages. As you will see, opportunities abound and creating an exhaustive list is all but impossible. View these lists as an inspirational starting point. Once again, if you do what you love, you will do it well, and this will help you get into medical school.

CLUBS

- ▶ Student government
- ▶ Model United Nations
- ▶ Debate club
- ▶ College democrats/republicans/independents
- ▶ Computer science society
- ▶ Writing club
- ▶ Literature/book club
- ▶ South Asian club
- ▶ Gaelic club
- ▶ Texas club
- ▶ Pre-med club
- ▶ Outdoors club
- ▶ Society for Muslim students
- ▶ Newman center (Catholic)
- ▶ Athletes in action
- ▶ WWJD club
- ▶ Hillel
- ▶ Meditation club
- ▶ Honors society
- ▶ Fraternities/sororities/secret societies

SPORTS

- ▶ Compete in NCAA division I, II, or III athletics
- ▶ Join club sports
- ▶ Play intramurals
- ▶ Race competitively (marathons, triathlons, cycling, rowing, *etc.*)
- ▶ Climb mountains
- ▶ Ski/snowboard
- ▶ Hike
- ▶ Kayak
- ▶ Whitewater raft
- ▶ Sail
- ▶ Surf
- ▶ Practice martial arts
- ▶ Perform yoga
- ▶ Play golf
- ▶ Ride/jump horses
- ▶ Coach athletics
- ▶ Serve as team manager
- ▶ Work as trainer
- ▶ Teach aerobics class
- ▶ Volunteer with Special Olympics

ARTS

- ► Act
- ► Direct
- ► Paint
- ► Draw
- ► Sculpt
- ► Photograph
- ► Design
- ► Dance
- ► Write
- ► Edit
- ► Blog
- ► Sing
- ► Knit/crochet
- ► Make jewelry
- ► Join newspaper
- ► Create yearbook
- ► Code websites
- ► Make maps
- ► Play an instrument
- ► Compose music

HOBBIES

- ► Cook
- ► Garden
- ► Play chess/cribbage/mahjong
- ► Fish
- ► Restore cars
- ► Fly airplanes
- ► Skydive
- ► Collect antiques
- ► Collect stamps/coins
- ► Collect art
- ► Collect vintage clothing
- ► Collect minerals/insects/fossils
- ► Collect comics/baseball cards
- ► Fix historic clocks
- ► Scrapbook
- ► Write computer programs
- ► Read science fiction
- ► Perform genealogy
- ► Woodwork
- ► Make model cars/airplanes/trains

TRAVEL

- ▶ Drive across country
- ▶ Backpack through Southeast Asia on $25 a day
- ▶ Tour Europe on Eurorail
- ▶ Visit US national parks
- ▶ Perform internship in Nigeria
- ▶ Collect musical instruments from around the world
- ▶ Watch a game at every major league baseball stadium
- ▶ Cycle across Ireland
- ▶ Volunteer at Olympic Games
- ▶ See favorite footballer at World Cup
- ▶ Visit ancestral homeland to complete family tree
- ▶ Spy the "big and little five" on safari in Africa
- ▶ Drive borrowed car through South America
- ▶ Keep travel blog
- ▶ Write for travel magazine
- ▶ Publish travel photos
- ▶ Learn how to "travel hack"
- ▶ Sail in the Caribbean
- ▶ Visit every major world desert
- ▶ Travel to all seven continents
- ▶ Climb the tallest mountain on each continent

LANGUAGES

- ▶ Travel to Costa Rica to learn Spanish
- ▶ Learn Mandarin through Rosetta Stone
- ▶ Teach Russian
- ▶ Study a new language for fun
- ▶ Take Arabic classes
- ▶ Join language club
- ▶ Meet language partner to practice French
- ▶ Study threatened languages
- ▶ Read all Harry Potter books in Spanish to improve language skills
- ▶ Learn Hebrew to communicate with family in Israel
- ▶ Study Hindu while working in India
- ▶ Take American Sign Language classes
- ▶ Read Italian literature
- ▶ Major in East Asians Studies
- ▶ Practice Urdu with parents
- ▶ Take semester abroad classes in another language
- ▶ Write a book in Portuguese
- ▶ Learn Korean by watching movies
- ▶ Work as German translator
- ▶ Study Persian poetry

OTHER

- ▶ Mentor
- ▶ Tutor/teach
- ▶ Peer counsel
- ▶ Consult
- ▶ Start a business
- ▶ Work/earn money
- ▶ Invest
- ▶ Be an apprentice
- ▶ Take a course
- ▶ Earn a Masters/PhD
- ▶ Lead a program
- ▶ Organize an event
- ▶ Build something
- ▶ Join a protest
- ▶ Start a movement
- ▶ Campaign for a candidate
- ▶ Run for office
- ▶ Adopt a pet
- ▶ Get married
- ▶ Raise children

As a medical school admissions consultant, I most enjoy hearing about my clients' extracurricular activities. It astounds me how frequently these pre-meds neglect to mention their favorite extracurriculars unless encouraged to do so. Do not underestimate their power. Extracurriculars often become useful parts of the AMCAS application's personal statement and work-activities sections. Additionally, they can often serve as a starting point for other activities, such as community service or research.

One of the best examples of using a hobby to springboard further activities comes from a former client. This young man, who I will call Dan, visited New York City and saw a group of elderly Chinese men playing Mahjong in the park. Enthralled with the game, he taught himself how to play upon returning home. Soon, he taught friends and started tournaments in the dorm. Realizing how invigorating he found the game, Dan decided to bring it to a local nursing home where he volunteered and often noticed the residents suffered from boredom and loneliness. Within months, the nursing home residents were fully engrossed in the game and engaged in competitive Mahjong tournaments organized by Dan. Why is this story about a Chinese table game so helpful for medical school admissions? Because Dan found something that interested him (shows curiosity), taught himself how to play it (shows self-motivation), taught the game to others (shows people skills), initiated tournaments among friends (shows leadership), and shared his love of the game with nursing home residents (shows creativity, compassion, and community building). This story, because of its uniqueness and ability to demonstrate so many of Dan's positive characteristics, comprised an entire paragraph of his medical school personal statement.

Do not ignore extracurriculars. You are about to enter a profession filled with considerable stress. Extracurricular activities are often the best way to blow off steam and stay grounded. Amidst the intense academic, research, community service, and clinical experience obligations of medical school admissions, remember to find time for yourself and to do the things you love.

MYTH BUSTERS: EXTRACURRICULARS
The pre-med rumor mill has created the following myths. All of these myths have been busted.
▸ Admissions committees don't care about extracurriculars. ▸ Every pre-med activity needs to directly relate to medicine or science. ▸ Extracurriculars are a waste of time. ▸ One-off extracurriculars are good enough for the medical school application. ▸ Extracurriculars are the least important part of the medical school application.

FILL IT UP

Use the area below to take notes on filling the Extracurriculars Bucket

CHAPTER 5

Clinical Experience

We have moved through the Academics, Research, Community Service, and Extracurriculars Buckets to arrive at the Clinical Experience Bucket. Clinical experience refers to any activity where you are learning the inner workings of doctorhood – from patient care to administrative headaches.

When speaking with members of medical school admissions committees, I continually hear, "Lack of clinical experience is the most common reason why pre-meds are not accepted to medical school." Not a low GPA or MCAT score. Not lackluster community service or research experience. It is insufficient clinical experience holding back many pre-meds. Let's think about this more – medical school admissions committees want to be sure you know what you are getting into. How can you be certain doctoring is your life calling if you never set foot in a hospital? Medicine is a hard path, as I am sure you have heard. How do you know you like taking care of sick people? How do you know medicine is the right profession for you? How do you know you can handle the pressures of being a doctor? The answer is simple – spend as much time with physicians and in medical settings as possible.

Here are some ways to gain clinical experience:

▸ Shadow physicians
▸ Volunteer in medical clinic/office/hospital/nursing home
▸ Work as scribe/EMT/paramedic/tech/phlebotomist
▸ Perform clinical research
▸ Travel on international medical mission
▸ Lifeguard
▸ Take BLS/ACLS/PALS/wilderness survival class
▸ Participate in disaster drill
▸ Be a patient
▸ Care for ill family/friends

Throughout this guide, I have reiterated how important it is to avoid one-offs. I am going to reverse this comment on one specific aspect of clinical experience – shadowing. Shadowing physicians and medical providers is a critical aspect of exploring the profession. Most doctors enjoy having a pre-med's excitement and energy around for a day or so. But few will appreciate a pre-med hanging around everyday. When it comes to shadowing physicians, breadth outweighs depth. For example, I think it is more important to spend a day each with five to 10 different doctors in different fields to gain experience with varying specialties, than to spend a month with one physician. If you have the opportunity to shadow multiple physicians for a prolonged period, go for it. But focus on getting a wide variety of experiences.

Imagine how much you will learn about medicine by spending a day shadowing an internist/primary care practitioner, pediatrician, general surgeon, neurologist, cardiologist, oncologist, radiologist, emergency physician, obstetrician/gynecologist, and ophthalmologist. More than anything, you will realize the medical profession offers incredible variety. If a particular specialty peaks your interest, feel free to explore it further through more shadowing or even research. But cast a wide net first and then narrow down your interests. When you refer to shadowing on the AMCAS application, list all of the experiences under one heading entitled, "Shadowing." No need to put a separate entry for each day you spent with a doctor.

Asking a physician for permission to shadow often leads to great anxiety for pre-meds. But there is no reason to be nervous. The worst the doctor can say is no. Some hospitals do not allow shadowing (mine, for example). But this is rare. When asking a physician for permission to shadow, simply pick up the phone and ask:

"Dr. Core, I am a pre-med at Maryland State University looking to gain more clinical experience. Would you mind if I spent a day shadowing you in the clinic?"

"Dr. Blade, I am a sophomore at District College on the pre-med track hoping to observe a few surgeries. Would it be possible for me to shadow you at the hospital and watch you perform surgeries?"

"Dr. Stat, I am a junior at Nebraska A&M very interested in a medical career. Would it be possible for me to shadow you during a emergency department shift?"

See? Asking a doctor for permission to shadow is not difficult.

Be clear who you are, why you want to shadow, and that you are only asking to visit for a day. If you cannot reach the doctor by phone, leave a voice mail. If your call is not returned in a week, feel free to send a follow-up e-mail. I suggest calling first as e-mails are often lost or forgotten. Be sure to write e-mails in a professional manner and avoid using slang or text-like abbreviations.

Don't know any physicians? Sure you do. Start with your own. Call up your primary care physician and ask to shadow him or her. Then ask this physician if he or she has any colleagues you could shadow. How about your relatives, parents' friends, parents' physicians, or friends' parents? Do they know any doctors? If you cannot come up with any physician references, check with your college's pre-med group or career service office and see if any mentoring programs exist where physicians have signed up. And if all else fails, hit the Internet. Look up doctors at your local hospital and start cold calling.

For the clinical experience options other than shadowing, it is best to focus on commitment and leadership, just as you have in research, community service, and extracurricular activities. For example, it is more impressive to spend four hours every Sunday volunteering in a nursing home, emergency department, or free clinic than just one day or one week. Because clinical experience is such an important part of medical school admissions, I suggest you spend as much time in a clinical setting as possible in addition to the shadowing experiences discussed above. It is often a good idea to obtain a reference from someone in the medical profession, and obtaining a long-term, regular, formal clinical experience is usually the best way to get to know a doctor who can write such a reference.

Since volunteering in a hospital, clinic, or nursing home is a very common way for pre-meds to gain clinical experience, most medical facilities have created volunteer programs. When looking for a clinical opportunity, I suggesting starting local. Call up the nearby hospital and ask for the volunteer coordinator. Most hospitals, clinics, and nursing homes will require you apply formally, commit to a minimum number of hours, and complete orientation.

When volunteering in a clinical environment, do not expect to save lives. You are not a doctor yet! Most volunteers spend their time performing menial tasks such as manning the information desk, fetching water and food for patients, cleaning beds, transporting patients, and organizing supplies. But while performing these simple jobs, you will witness how medicine really works – the teamwork required to perform surgery, the importance of nursing to patient care, the long waits and frustration many patients face, the mixture of fear and joy so common in the hospital, and the many obstacles physicians confront when trying to care for patients. Your job while volunteering is to perform the given tasks while acting like a sponge, soaking up every detail of what it is like to care for sick people all day, every day.

One way to get more involved in the clinical realm is to work in a clinical setting. There are quite a few jobs available to pre-meds that allow patient contact after obtaining requisite training. For example, medical scribes are becoming more common in the hospital setting. Scribes literally shadow physicians during their shifts in the hospital or office and then create the medical chart. The pay is not stellar, but working as a scribe is a wonderful way to learn the language of medicine and intimately witness the inner workings of doctorhood. Serving as an emergency medical technician (EMT) allows you to directly care for patients in the pre-hospital setting. Classes are required but can frequently be completed during evenings or summers. If you enjoy working as an EMT, consider becoming a paramedic. Note the transition from EMT to paramedic requires considerable training because paramedics are able to answer the most complex emergency medical system (EMS) calls and perform difficult procedures. Many hospitals and clinics hire EMTs as "techs" responsible for obtaining vitals, drawing blood, performing electrocardiograms (EKGs), placing splints, and assisting with cardiopulmonary resuscitation (CPR). Another way to get involved with direct patient care is to become a phlebotomist, or someone who specializes in drawing blood. All of these jobs offer more direct patient contact compared to volunteer or shadowing positions.

Even more opportunities exist in the clinical realm. You can join a clinical research team, travel on a medical mission abroad, or work as a lifeguard. If you are limited in time, consider medical classes such basic life support (BLS), advanced cardiac life support (ACLS), pediatric advanced life support (PALS), or wilderness medicine. Disaster preparedness groups often run disaster drills and are always looking for volunteers. Even if you are not in the hospital setting, you can still gain clinical experience.

Many pre-meds first gain interest in medicine because of a personal illness or caring for a sick loved one. These experiences can be profound and often life changing and certainly can be included in the medical school application. In fact, such experiences often make for excellent anecdotes in the AMCAS personal statement.

I cannot emphasize enough the importance of gaining clinical experience as a pre-med. This is something you should do early and often. What if you do not enjoy being around sick people? That is great! You have avoided years of difficult training and financial cost (both actual and opportunity cost). Remember, you should only become a doctor if there is nothing else in the world you can imagine doing. It is a wonderful profession, but it is not for everybody. So go find out if it is the right profession for you by spending as much time as possible in the clinical environment.

MYTH BUSTERS: CLINICAL EXPERIENCE
The pre-med rumor mill has created the following myths. All of these myths have been busted.
▸ Clinical experience is not an essential part of the medical school application. ▸ You have to shadow a physician for weeks for it to count. ▸ Volunteering in the emergency department for a few weeks provides plenty of clinical experience. ▸ All clinical experience must occur in the hospital. ▸ Pre-meds can never find opportunities to work directly with patients. ▸ Being a patient and caring for an ill loved one are not significant clinical experiences.

FILL IT UP

Use the area below to take notes on filling
the Clinical Experience Bucket

CHAPTER 6

Application Skills

We have made it to the sixth and final bucket: Application Skills. Once you have earned stellar grades, aced the MCAT, and obtained meaningful, long-term research, community service, extracurricular, and clinical experiences, there is still more work to be done. The medical school admissions process is easily the most difficult and complicated when compared to other types of graduate school applications. It seems the admissions committees do this on purpose. Given the demands of medical school, residency, and doctoring, admissions committees use the grueling application process to prevent all but those certain of their desire to become physicians from applying. Medical school does not have an, "I'll just apply and see what happens" kind of application process.

According to the AAMC, 43,919 pre-meds applied to medical school in 2011. 19,230 matriculated. Thus, less than 44% of pre-meds who applied were accepted and matriculated to medical school. I never cease to be amazed how many exceptional pre-meds exist today and how the competition to get into medical school seems to increase over time. But having helped pre-meds gain acceptance to medical school for over a decade, I have seen stellar candidates originally rejected and mediocre pre-meds get in. Why? Because it takes more than excellent grades, research, community service, extracurricular, and clinical experiences to get into medical school. You can do everything "right," and then write a poor application that results in rejection. This is why the Application Skills Bucket is just as important as the last five buckets, and why I wrote *The Medical School Admissions Guide: A Harvard MD's Week-by-Week Admissions Handbook* dedicated to helping pre-meds excel in the application process. Application skills are often the difference between acceptance and rejection by medical school admissions committees.

Pick up *The Medical School Admissions Guide* (available online at Amazon, Barnes and Noble, and MDadmit.com) by January of your application year. Though you do not need to know every detail in the Guide until you decide to apply, understanding application basics early in your pre-med years will give you an advantage. Thus, I use this chapter to lay out the medical school application steps and show you how to start working on the application years before you actually submit it.

The Story

Getting into medical school requires telling a compelling story. Each aspect of the application should coalesce into a unique narrative helping you stand out among the other over 40,000 applicants and persuading the medical school admissions committees of your ability to become an excellent physician.

When composing your own story, think about what you would

tell an admissions committee member during a short elevator ride. This "elevator pitch" is not your whole narrative, but provides a starting point as you develop the story's theme. Here are compelling elevator pitches from some of my clients who became successful medical school applicants:

> ▸ Junior in large public university inspired by grandfather's 40-year career as family practitioner who confirmed importance of medicine's personal side through serving as EMT, Big Brother, and clinical research assistant.

> ▸ Forty-year-old software developer returned to pre-med post-baccalaureate courses after caring for friends dying of AIDS and subsequently worked as HIV counselor, developed software for free clinic, and performed psychiatric research. He hopes to become internist or psychiatrist working with patients suffering from chronic disease.

> ▸ First generation Sri Lankan who became interested in ophthalmology as a child requiring glasses and pursued interest through participating in free eye clinics for disadvantaged inner city populations, performing ophthalmology research, and founding sustainable eye clinic in Sri Lanka.

> ▸ MD/PhD candidate whose interest in research started while teaching music to autistic child and who used patience, thoughtful reflection, and communication skills practiced as singer to advance scientific investigations.

▶ African-American woman who attended traditionally black college, served in sorority and club leadership roles, worked in free clinic serving indigent minority patients, and wants to become primary care physician concentrating on decreasing health disparities in black communities.

▶ Captain of Harvard basketball team who became interested in medicine when teammate tore ACL and now desires to become orthopedic surgeon to help others maintain mobility and athletic prowess.

▶ Engineering major who cared for bipolar sister and wishes to use analytic skills to improve evidence base of psychiatric field.

▶ Cancer survivor who created video games to help child cancer patients understand importance of taking medicine, researched environmental impact on cancer development, and now aims to become oncologic surgeon.

▶ Philosophy major who wrote undergraduate thesis on ethics, interned in biomedical ethics, and hopes to work as clinician who contributes to field of bioethics.

▶ Asian woman with masters in public health who spent two years working in free clinic and studying relationship between poverty and disease and wants to become a primary care physician delivering care to disadvantaged communities.

- Visual arts major who used art therapy to help poverty-stricken children suffering from chronic diseases in South America and now seeks to become physician embracing both art and science of medicine to best treat patients.

- Indian immigrant with permanent US residency who spent four years studying basic science of colon cancer and wishes to pursue MD/PhD degree with oncology focus.

- Army officer who became interested in medicine during active duty in Iraq where she watched military doctors provide excellent care to both US soldiers and enemy combatants, gained clinical experience both in and out of the military, and wants to become physician who provides compassionate care to those most in need regardless of background.

- Jewish man who dedicated free time to volunteering in Jewish nursing home and serving in synagogue and desires to become primary care physician for New York City's Orthodox communities.

- Government major who spent two years working as health policy research assistant and aims to pursue MD/MPP degree to then serve as internist and health policy expert.

- Lesbian who volunteered in clinic assisting transgender individuals, interned in a reproductive and sexual health foundation, and aspires to become endocrinologist that runs transgender clinic.

- Medical engineering major who developed automatic straw device for paraplegics' wheelchairs and clean water systems for Central American community and wants to become physician who works clinically and creates appropriate medical devices for developing world.

- Recent college graduate who cared for mother during breast cancer treatment, volunteered at breast cancer foundation, performed laboratory research on cancer-causing genes, and now wishes to become oncologist.

- Behavioral science major who performed research on how behavior affects diabetes treatment and wants to help patients with chronic disease change behavior to lead healthy life.

- Man of Irish descent who grew up in Texas, learned Spanish in school, volunteered with disadvantaged border communities, and traveled on multiple medical missions to Central and South America who aspires to become a primary care physician serving Spanish-speaking immigrants.

> ▸ Lawyer who returned to post-baccalaureate pre-med studies after working for legal aid helping indigent clients suffering from chronic health conditions, volunteered in free clinic, performed policy research on health insurance options for the poor, and now hopes to become a doctor assisting with both medical and social issues faced by disadvantaged communities.
>
> ▸ Junior in college with interest in cardiothoracic surgery who worked in surgical research lab, volunteered in surgical intensive care unit, and shadowed over ten different surgeons.

As you can see from these examples, successful medical school applications may be filled with a wide variety of stories. No one particular story guarantees acceptance to medical school. The key is to be true to yourself and create a narrative supported by life experiences. Though every research, community service, extracurricular, and clinical activity need not directly relate to your story's theme, an overarching narrative must exist. I suggest contemplating how to weave your interests into a compelling story early in the pre-med process.

You may worry about the specificity of the above examples. How did these pre-meds know precisely what they wanted to do with the rest of their lives? In general, they did not know exactly. But these pre-meds did have an inkling, an interest, or a leaning allowing them to describe what kind of doctor they would like to be. Notice every story does not name an specific specialty. It is often enough to discuss the general population you want to care for or how you hope to include other interests like research, policy, ethics, global health, engineering, art, or design.

Medical school admissions committees will not check back in four years to see if you stuck with the story. The narrative theme I used in the medical school application is included above – "Captain of Harvard basketball team who became interested in medicine when teammate tore ACL and now desires to become orthopedic surgeon to help others maintain mobility and athletic prowess." But after doing an orthopedic rotation in medical school, I decided orthopedics involved a bit more hammering and drilling than I liked. Since I still wanted a fast-paced, team-oriented profession where I could use my hands, sharpen diagnostic skills, and work internationally, I became an emergency physician. But at application time, I wanted to be an orthopedist and created a strong narrative supported by life-experiences in sports, community service, and clinical activities to show the medical school admissions committees why I would be an excellent medical student and physician.

Every pre-med has a story. What is yours? As we move through the medical school application's specific steps, we will follow five pre-meds to see how they created a compelling narrative. Though their stories differ greatly, all five gained admissions to top medical schools. As you read the narratives of Tyler, Kevin, Padma, Mary, and Gabbi, keep in mind how each aspect of the application can be used to help create your story. Of course, Tyler, Kevin, Padma, Mary, and Gabbi are not these pre-meds' actual names. I have changed all names, dates, and personal information to protect their identities. These changes lead to generalized statements, such as "in the Caribbean," or "a university." When writing your application, you, of course, want to be as specific as possible. Before exploring our pre-meds' narratives, a further explanation of the admissions process is necessary.

AMCAS Application

In the old days, every US medical school had its own unique application. Fortunately, the American Association of Medical Colleges (AAMC) created the American Medical College Application Service (AMCAS) to run one primary application for virtually all allopathic medical schools. AMCAS does not make the admissions decisions, but instead serves as a centralized application processor. It is up to each medical school's admissions committee to determine if you get in or not. Public medical schools in Texas (TMD-SAS), osteopathic medical schools (AACOMAS), and Canadian medical schools in Ontario Province (OMSAS) all have centralized applications separate from AMCAS. To make things more confusing, some Texas schools' MD/PhD programs use AMCAS, while schools in Canadian provinces other than Ontario and off-shore/foreign schools each have their own individual applications. Before you apply, check which schools and programs use which service. See the box "Important Application Websites" for links to each centralized application.

IMPORTANT APPLICATION WEBSITES	
AMCAS	https://www.aamc.org/students/applying/amcas/
TMDSAS	http://www.utsystem.edu/tmdsas/
AACOMAS	http://aacomas.aacom.org/
OMSAS	http://www.ouac.on.ca/omsas/ (rest of Canadian schools have individual applications)

Please note the term allopathic generally refers to medical schools teaching "mainstream" or "Western" medicine and offering a MD degree. Interestingly, Samuel Hahnemann, the founder of homeopathic medicine, coined "allopathic" in 1810 as a pejorative term. Osteopathic medical schools offer a DO degree and teach both Western medical concepts and manipulative therapy such as chiropracty. Both MD and DO degrees provide an opportunity to practice medicine in the United States. Historically, the MD degree has been viewed as more prestigious. But the DO degree is gaining interest because of the osteopathic emphasis on treating the "whole" patient and incorporating alternative medical practices. In general, DO programs are less competitive than MD programs, but gaining acceptance to an osteopathic medical school is becoming more competitive every year. The rest of this section will focus on applying to allopathic medical schools in the US. Please see *The Medical School Admissions Guide* for more information on osteopathic, offshore, and foreign school options.

AMCAS starts accepting applications in June even though medical school deadlines range from October to December. If you want to start medical school in the fall of 2014, you should submit the AMCAS in June of 2013. Submitting the application early is of paramount importance because rolling admissions schools offer secondary applications, interviews, and acceptances on a first-come, first-served basis. Many pre-meds have been foiled by October AMCAS submissions because most schools have already offered all of their interview invites by then. The moral of this story – apply as early as possible.

Unfortunately, the AMCAS application (https://www.aamc.org/students/applying/amcas/) is generally not available online until April or May of any given year. For example, the application for matriculation in fall of 2014 will be made available in April or May of 2013. When your goal is to submit the AMCAS in June, this does not seem to leave much time. Fortunately, you can start preparing for the AMCAS application much earlier as the application basics tend to remain the same from year to year. The AAMC creates a downloadable instruction manual on the AMCAS webpage providing detailed information on how to complete the application and highlighting any changes from previous years. It also provides an application worksheet allowing you to begin entering application information on paper before the official online version is available. These resources can be found at https://www.aamc.org/students/applying/amcas/amcasresources/. Both the manual and application worksheets are must-reads before you apply.

To officially start the medical school application process, register online at https://www.aamc.org/students/applying/amcas/ to create an AAMC username and password. Then you can enter the online application and start adding information. Until you hit the final submit button, you can save details and return to make changes. We will move through the AMCAS application's eight sections now, highlighting when you can start preparing for each part and showing how to use the application to create a story.

AMCAS Section I: Identifying Information

Luckily, the AMCAS application starts off easy. In the first AMCAS section, you are asked to provide identifying information including formal name, nickname, social security number, birthday, and sex.

AMCAS Section II: Schools Attended

The AMCAS application is quite picky when it comes to schools attended. It requires you provide information on your high school and has special instructions if you were home schooled, received a General Education Development (GED) certification, or attended high school in another country. Then it asks you to list all post-high school educational institutions attended, even if you withdrew, transferred course credit, or did not receive credit from these schools. AMCAS includes community college, summer school, and study abroad programs in this definition. You cannot hide from any post-secondary courses taken because AMCAS requires transcripts from every post-secondary institution attended. Using the AMCAS Transcript Request Form found inside the AMCAS application, you can ask your registrar(s) to send an official transcript directly to AMCAS. Request an extra transcript for yourself to help complete the coursework section of the application.

In the Schools Attended section, you will also be asked about previous matriculation into medical school and any institutional action filed against you. Medical schools take institutional action very seriously. The worst thing you can do is withhold information and have the medical school admissions committees find out about an incident later – this will undoubtedly lead to a rejection even if you have already been accepted into medical school. As stated on the AAMC's AMCAS webpage, any "academic performance or a conduct violation, even if such action did not interrupt your enrollment, require you to withdraw, or does not appear on your official transcripts due to institutional policy or personal petition" must be acknowledged and explained. When writing about such experiences, it is best to be brief. In 1325 characters or less, describe what happened and what you learned from it. Admissions committees do not want to read lengthy sob stories. I have seen many applicants thwarted by institutional action regarding illegal use of alcohol while underage. Hopefully knowing the strictness of AMCAS' rules will be added incentive for you to make good decisions.

AMCAS Section III: Biographical Information

Section III of the AMCAS application requests your biographic information, such as address, phone number, e-mail, citizenship, legal residence (which is important if you are applying to state schools), languages spoken, and race/ethnicity. AMCAS communicates mainly via e-mail, so be sure to input a valid e-mail address you will use for the next year.

This section also offers a chance to determine if you qualify for "disadvantaged status." You will be required to provide parents'/guardians' level of education and current employment information, number and age of siblings, family's income, and information about how you paid for college. In addition, you are allowed 1325 characters to answer the question, "Do you believe you have faced any hardships from birth to present that interfered with your educational pursuits?" Many medical schools are moving their affirmative action policies away from assessing race and ethnicity to a more comprehensive evaluation of a candidate's access to opportunities. If you come from a disadvantaged background, do not be ashamed to admit it. "Disadvantaged" does not refer only to racial or ethnic status because the economic, familial, and geographic details of your upbringing may also play a role. Medical school admissions committees take disadvantaged status very seriously and often give applicants who have overcome barriers an advantage in the application process. If you are unsure whether or not you meet disadvantaged status criteria, speak with your college's premed advisor or a medical school admissions consultant who can help guide you. And if you do have a disadvantaged story to tell, this is your first opportunity to weave it into the overall application narrative.

In addition, the Biographical Information section requests you disclose and explain any misdemeanors or felonies. Interestingly, the AMCAS application also states that if you "are convicted of, plead guilty, or no contest to a felony or misdemeanor crime, you must inform the admissions office of each medical school to which you have applied" if the event occurs after the submissions date. I know of multiple pre-meds accepted into medical school and then convicted of driving while under the influence of alcohol or possession of marijuana. Every medical school subsequently withdrew acceptances. Even after you press the AMCAS submission button or receive a letter of acceptance, you are still obligated to be a law-abiding citizen.

AMCAS Section IV: Coursework

Be sure to have your official transcripts handy when filling out AMCAS' Coursework section. For every school you have attended after high school, you will be asked to provide academic status, course number, course name, course classification, course type, credit hours, and official transcript grade. Once you have entered the data, the AMCAS system will automatically generate your GPA and break it down into:

- Cumulative GPA
- Science GPA (*i.e.*, BCPM – biology, chemistry, physics, and math)
- All Other GPA (AO)

Remember, you have to enter every course taken post high school, even if no credit was earned. AMCAS even wants to see "courses removed from your transcripts or GPA as a result of academic bankruptcy, forgiveness, or similar institutional policies." They are tough! The only courses that do not count towards to AMCAS GPA are pass/fail – pass, pass/fail – fail, advanced placement (AP) credit, College Level Examination Program (CLEP) credit, audited courses, and courses officially withdrawn or "dropped." AMCAS reports the total hours for these first four types of courses under a "Supplementary Hours" heading.

AMCAS verifies every course based on your official transcript and calculates GPAs prior to transmitting applications to medical schools. Of note, AMCAS often generates different GPAs than many undergraduate institutions because it counts virtually every course and has a standard calculation for "+" and "-" grades. In general, AMCAS GPAs are a tad lower than transcript grades. Rarely have I seen a GPA change by more than one tenth unless the AMCAS counts a course with a poor grade that a pre-med's university did not.

Here are Tyler's grades as AMCAS presents them to medical schools:

Status	BCPM		AO		Total	
	GPA	Hours	GPA	Hours	GPA	Hours
High School						
Freshman	3.47	17.00	2.75	12.00	3.17	29.00
Sophomore	3.32	19.00	4.00	18.00	3.65	37.00
Junior	3.77	22.00	4.00	6.00	3.82	28.00
Senior	3.75	24.00			3.75	24.00
Postbaccalaureate Undergraduate						
Cumulative Undergraduate	3.60	82.00	3.58	36.00	3.59	118.00
Graduate	4.00	4.00			4.00	4.00
Supplemental Hours	**P/F – Pass: 2.00**	**P/F – Fail:**	**A/P: 39.00**	**CLEP:**	**OTHER: 2.00**	

Entering course classification and study abroad classes often causes great confusion for pre-meds. Remember the "Course Classification Guide" from the Academics Bucket that helped you figure out which courses counted for pre-med requirements? Get it out again (you can find it at https://www.aamc.org/students/download/181694/data/amcas_course_classification_guide.pdf). In addition, the AMCAS instruction manual (https://www.aamc.org/students/download/182162/data/amcas_instruction_manual.pdf) addresses when and how to enter study abroad and foreign courses. In general, if study abroad credits were transferred to a US institution, you do not need a separate transcript from the foreign school and must enter the courses exactly as they appear on your US college transcript.

AMCAS Section V: Work/Activities

Now we are entering the meat of the medical school application where your narrative will come into better focus. Think of the AMCAS work/activities section as an annotated resume. Here you can show the medical school admissions committees your impressive research, community service, extracurricular, and clinical experiences. As of 2011, AMCAS modified the work/activities section requirements, allowing 15 work/activity entries of 700 characters plus three "most meaningful" activities out of those listed with additional 1325 characters of explanation.

AMCAS categorizes work/activities entries as follows:

- Paid Employment – Not Military
- Paid Employment – Military
- Community Service/Volunteer – Not Medical/Clinical
- Community Service/Volunteer – Medical/Clinical
- Research/Lab
- Publications
- Presentations/Posters
- Conferences Attended
- Teaching/Tutoring
- Intercollegiate Athletics
- Extracurricular/Hobbies/Avocations
- Honors/Awards/Recognition
- Leadership – Not Listed Elsewhere
- Other

AMCAS requests you include experience type, experience name, experience dates, average hours per week, organization name, country, city, and the name, title, phone number, and e-mail of a contact that can vouch you participated in the activity. This contact may be a professor, coach, community service advisor, principal investigator, *etc*. It should not be a member of your family. If the activity relates to a student-organized group with no advisor, you may list a contact in your university's student affairs office to verify participation. If absolutely no contact is known, you can enter a peer or yourself. Use this option as a last resort.

When filling out the work/activities section, only include significant experiences and avoid repeats. For example, if you shadowed multiple physicians for one day each, create one "shadowing" entry and list the details of each shadowing experience. You can also put all awards and publications under one entry. Aim to compose an easy-to-read AMCAS work/activities section in the same way you would create a resume. Medical school admissions committee members often breeze through this section quickly. Do note AMCAS automatically lists work/activities entries in chronological order, which may not be rearranged by you. The admissions committees can sort the work/activities section in any order they choose.

There is no need to fill all 15 entries. I rarely allow clients 15 work/activities because, frankly, few pre-meds have 15 exceptional experiences. Medical school admissions committees prefer to see nine stellar work/activities entries rather than 15 mediocre ones.

Many pre-meds struggle with which three activities to mark as "most meaningful." Remember the story theme I have been harping on? It comes into play again here. Which three activities best fit into your overall narrative? Which three highlight your well-rounded skills? Which three are most likely to prove to admissions committees you will be an exceptional medical student and physician? Be careful picking three similar activities. For example, it is usually best to choose one research, one extracurricular, and one clinical experience activity as opposed to three research activities. According to AMCAS, "When writing your ["most meaningful" activity] response, you might want to consider the transformative nature of the experience, the impact you made while engaging in the activity, and the personal growth you experienced as a result of your participation." I suggest using the initial 700 characters to describe the experience and the following 1325 characters to highlight how this activity affected your life. While writing these "most meaningful" narratives, always consider how they relate to your overall story.

There is no more powerful way to learn how to best complete an activity than to see an excellent example. So let us read and evaluate how Tyler, Kevin, Padma, Mary, and Gabbi filled out their AMCAS work/activities sections. As you read these examples, notice the narrative each is beginning to tell. What themes do you pick up from each work/activities section example? Do you agree with the most meaningful activities choices? Are they telling you a story? Do not concentrate on every detail of the AMCAS work/activity examples. They can be densely packed with specifics. Instead play the role of an admissions committee member and quickly read through each taking in the overall message.

To maintain privacy, I have removed or changed all personal information from these AMCAS work/activity examples including contact name and title, contact e-mail, organization name, and city/state/country. Don't forget this information will be required when you fill out the AMCAS work/activities section. I have also changed any specifics, including names of people and institutions, research references, and locations to maintain author privacy.

Example 1: Tyler's AMCAS Work/Activities

Tyler's admissions elevator pitch:

> *Junior in large public university inspired by grandfather's 40-year career as family practitioner who confirmed importance of medicine's personal side through serving as EMT, Big Brother, and clinical research assistant.*

Though Taylor's elevator pitch mentions serving as an EMT, Big Brother, and clinical research assistant, he does not choose all three of these as most meaningful experiences. He uses EMT and clinical research as most meaningful activities but selects playing college lacrosse as his third. I think this is a good move on Tyler's part. Because his lacrosse experience does not fit well into the personal statement (as you will see in the Essays Section), he highlights remarkable determination and leadership qualities through choosing lacrosse as one of his most meaningful entries. Though it is acceptable to make your three most meaningful activities the same as in your personal statement, this does not always have to be the case.

Experience Type: Community Service/Volunteer – Medical/Clinical
Most Meaningful Experience: No
Experience Name: Preceptorship
Dates: 08/2012 – 12/2012
Hours/Week: 8
Experience Description: I shadowed Dr. Leary, a primary care physician, one day a week for five months. Dr. Leary has practiced in his current private clinic for 26 years and offered me a chance to

meet a wide-variety of patients, witness the inner-workings of a busy private practice, and learn the importance of every member of the medical team. Observing the deep relationships Dr. Leary has formed with many of his patients only increased my desire to become a physician dedicated to treating the whole patient.

Experience Type: Community Service/Volunteer – Medical/Clinical
Most Meaningful Experience: No
Experience Name: Hospice Volunteer
Dates: 08/2010 – Until Present
Hours/Week: 5
Experience Description: I have served as a hospice patient caregiver and aid for the past three years. My role includes socializing with patients and assisting with everyday activities such as shopping and cooking. I also provide support to families who are helping care for family members in hospice. Taking part in end-of-life care has increased my comfort caring for those with dire illnesses and solidified my belief in the importance of dying with dignity.

Experience Type: Research/Lab
Most Meaningful Experience: Yes
Experience Name: Chief Research Assistant
Dates: 05/2010 – Until Present
Hours/Week: 14
Experience Description: I serve as chief research assistant to Dr. Bert Callahan on an investigation of ilio-tibial band surgical techniques. Past research included reading medical journals and participating in multiple cadaver dissections, where I measured ilio-tibial band insertions into the gluteus maximus. Future research includes monitoring pressure changes due to various incisions along the

band. Recently, I co-authored an abstract for potential publication with the American Association of Orthopedic Surgeons.

Most Meaningful Experience Remarks: Dr. Callahan has integrated me fully into his research team. I thrive on the challenge of using both mental and physical tools to answer a hypothetical research question and enjoy seeing the possible real-life effects of our research. I have enjoyed every step of the research process from literature searches to data gathering to abstract creation and look forward to seeing a project through from start to publication. I hope to continue contributing to research throughout medical school and beyond. Working as a chief research assistant has only increased my desire to become a physician who cures patients using techniques rigorously tested in the laboratory setting.

Experience Type: Community Service/Volunteer – Medical/Clinical
Most Meaningful Experience: No
Experience Type: Research/Lab
Most Meaningful Experience: No
Experience Name: Chief Research Assistant
Dates: 05/2010 – 08/2010
Hours/Week: 18
Experience Description: I served as the chief assistant on a study of hip resurfacing surgical techniques that involved a retrospective review of over 400 patient files, surgical reports, and x-rays. Research included charting patient progress through improvements in Hip Harris Score. Currently, a data summary is being compiled for presentation at an orthopedic conference in the coming months.

Experience Type: Extracurricular/Hobbies/Avocations
Most Meaningful Experience: No

Experience Name: Triathlons
Dates: 03/2010 – Until Present
Hours/Week: 8
Experience Description: I have participated in three sprint triathlons and continue to enter triathlons each summer. Training includes daily running, swimming, and biking, and this exercise serves as a period of relaxation. Along with triathlons, I have begun training for a marathon and hope to complete my first 26.2-mile race in February with a goal of finishing in less than 4 hours.

Experience Type: Leadership – Not Listed Elsewhere
Most Meaningful Experience: No
Experience Name: Pan-Hellenic Olympics Chairman
Dates: 05/2009 – 12/2009
Hours/Week: 12
Experience Description: As chairman, I planned a Pan-Hellenic sporting event raising over $1,600 for the American Cancer Society. My role also included collaboration with alumni, sponsors, and participants. This position allowed me to combine my passion for sports and helping others while honing leadership skills.

Experience Type: Other
Most Meaningful Experience: Yes
Experience Name: Emergency Medical Technician
Dates: 05/2008 – 08/2008
Hours/Week: 50
Experience Description: I enrolled in Emergency Medical Technician Basic training following freshman year. The course consisted of 25 hours of classroom training and 25 hours of skills training per week. Following classroom instruction, my certification includ-

ed four hospital rotations and two ambulance rotations that produced valuable clinical experience.

Most Meaningful Experience Remarks: Training as an Emergency Medical Technician (EMT) was pivotal in my decision to pursue medicine. The opportunity to treat my first patients was both thrilling and anxiety provoking. One initial call involved a motorcyclist in a highway-speed accident who required transfer to the trauma center via helicopter. I bagged the patient with oxygen while we transported him to the helicopter site. It was invigorating to use technical skills to contribute positively to another's health. With each medic call, I gained confidence while practicing bedside manner. Now that I have obtained basic EMT skills, I am eager to expand my medical knowledge to help those affected by trauma and illness and develop deeper relationships with patients.

Experience Type: Community Service/Volunteer – Not Medical/Clinical
Most Meaningful Experience: No
Experience Name: Big Brother
Dates: 01/2008 – 05/2011
Hours/Week: 2
Experience Description: My role with the program spanned two and a half years with the same "little brother." I guided him both academically and socially as he graduated from elementary school and entered the hectic middle school environment. During the mentorship, academic tutoring led to a significant increase in his grades. But most importantly, we molded a strong friendship I hope will continue long into the future.

Experience Type: Intercollegiate Athletics
Most Meaningful Experience: Yes
Experience Name: University Lacrosse
Dates: 01/2008 – 03/2010
Hours/Week: 15
Experience Description: I played lacrosse in both fall and spring semesters. We practiced for eight hours a week and played an average of two games per weekend. I finished my career second on the school's all-time points scored list, completed the 2009 season with the fifth highest assists per game in the nation, and was voted the team's most outstanding attackman in 2009. I was one of three team co-captains chosen by teammates and coaches and was the only underclassmen captain elected.

Most Meaningful Experience Remarks: I learned a great deal about commitment, loss, exhilaration, dedication, and pain from sports. Sophomore year, my commitment was tested by numerous team losses on the field, several injuries, and a heavily loaded academic schedule. Toward the end of the season, we experienced a season-changing moment. Losing decisively with 18 seconds left in the game, I stepped into the path of a defender to fire a shot and scored. I was leveled by the defenseman, but the moment was worth the pain. The scoreboard disparity remained, but it was a turning point for our team – we would fight to the very end, even if only for pride. After that game, the "never give up" spirit served as inspiration. With new resolve, we won the next four games, enjoying our first winning season in over six years. I am confident the tenacity sharpened on the field will prove instrumental in my career, as I face the inevitable challenges of medicine and use leadership skills to inspire my care team and patients.

My experience in lacrosse has demonstrated that determination can be contagious.

Experience Type: Community Service/Volunteer – Medical/Clinical
Most Meaningful Experience: No
Experience Name: Emergency Department Volunteer
Dates: 01/2008 – 10/2008
Hours/Week: 7
Experience Description: I served as a patient liaison and communicated patient concerns and questions to doctors and nurses. My position also included assisting and comforting patients during their stay in the emergency department. In the sole Level I Trauma Center in the region, I witnessed multiple trauma cases and enjoyed observing the teamwork so critical to success in the trauma bay.

Experience Name: Shadowing
Dates: 12/2007 – 07/2010
Hours/Week: 8
Experience Type: Other
Experience Description: To gain a deeper understanding of the surgical field, I shadowed a liver transplant and orthopedic surgeon. Dr. Eisenberg has practiced medicine for over 25 years and served as a wonderful teacher. I witnessed the high stakes and stressful days consistently encountered by surgeons. I also had the chance to watch a liver transplant surgery and attend the transplant meeting discussing potential surgical candidates. Previously, I observed several orthopedic surgeries with Dr. Rice, including a hip replacement and resurfacing and total knee arthroplasty, and attended post-op follow-up visits with these same patients.

Example 2: Kevin's AMCAS Work/Activities

Kevin's admissions elevator pitch:

Forty-year-old software developer returned to pre-med post-baccalaureate courses after caring for friends dying of AIDS and subsequently worked as HIV counselor, developed software for free clinic, and performed psychiatric research. He hopes to become internist or psychiatrist working with patients suffering from chronic disease.

What I love most about Kevin's AMCAS work/activities is how he epitomizes doing what you love and doing it well. He only lists eight activities. And yet he has one of the strongest work/activities sections I have ever seen. You can tell he used a life-changing experience (taking care of friends dying of AIDS) to spur healthcare exploration and a passion for clinical care and research.

Experience Type: Research/Lab
Most Meaningful Experience: Yes
Experience Name: Research Assistant
Dates: 10/2010 – 12/2011
Hours/Week: 5-20
Experience Description: I joined a psychology laboratory to further my interest in the social function and physiological basis of emotions. I started on a project examining the emotional functioning of patients with Alzheimer's disease and frontotemporal lobar degeneration (FTLD), and then became lead research assistant on a study of linguistic patterns in patients with dementia. I was also part of a team analyzing heterosexual, lesbian, and gay couples'

communication patterns and physiological responses during stressful conversations. While working in the lab, I participated in weekly lab meetings and literature reviews.

Most Meaningful Experience Remarks: This was my first substantial clinical research experience and provided an excellent introduction to the interaction between emotions and health. While studying the emotional functioning of patients with Alzheimer's disease and FTLD, I helped guide subjects through a series of emotion-inducing tasks (such as recalling their wedding day) while recording physiological reactions, facial expressions, and subjective experience. After six months in the lab, I received a promotion to lead research assistant on a study of linguistic patterns in dementia patients. We measured the degree to which patients' language reflected a connection to bodily and emotional experience, looking for linguistic patterns that might provide subtle signs of dementia onset and possibly serve as the basis for an inexpensive screening tool. During this project, I coordinated the activities of other research assistants and wrote computer programs to help analyze patients' memories of significant events (like JFK's assassination). I enjoyed every aspect of clinical research, from the individual interaction with each research subject to data analysis to manuscript creation.

Experience Type: Community Service/Volunteer – Medical/Clinical
Most Meaningful Experience: Yes
Experience Name: HIV Counselor/Clinic Assistant
Dates: 06/2009 – Present
Hours/Week: 4
Experience Description: Motivated by caring for friends dying of AIDS in the 1990s, I have become a certified HIV Counselor providing pre- and post-test HIV counseling to a high-risk population

at a community-based clinic. I conduct individual counseling sessions including risk assessment, discussion of harm reduction goals, motivational interviewing, preparation of harm-reduction plans, and referrals to primary care, mental health, and substance abuse services. I administer HIV tests and give test results, both positive and negative.

Most Meaningful Experience Remarks: During this counseling experience, I have been challenged by difficult discussions with individuals who want to contract HIV, adults afraid of any sexual contact for fear of infection, minors engaging in unprotected sex with adults, and clients afraid to tell partners of their status. In addition to active counseling, I participate in regular continuing education activities. I also perform STD testing for symptomatic and asymptomatic clients, run routine laboratory tests, and administer STD treatment. Working one-on-one with individuals struggling with the effects of a chronic disease confirmed my desire to enter medicine.

Experience Type: Community Service/Volunteer – Medical/Clinical
Most Meaningful Experience: Yes
Experience Name: Designer/Programmer: Electronic Medical Record and Case Management System/Clinic Assistant
Dates: 05/2009 – Present
Hours/Week: 7
Experience Description: I volunteered at an acute care clinic and community center acting as a "point of entry" and health care system guide to a mostly immigrant population. As clinic assistant, I took patients' vital signs, ran routine laboratory tests, performed immunizations and PPDs, filled prescriptions, and processed referrals to primary care, social service, and mental health providers. Seeing an opportunity to use my programming skills to benefit the

clinic, I now serve as one of two principal developers of a web-based medical record and case management system.

Most Meaningful Experience Remarks: Volunteering at the clinic provided a window into the difficult medical problems faced by immigrants and disadvantaged populations and allowed me to follow patients with various diseases including diabetes, COPD, work-related fractures, severe skin infections, depression, and high blood pressure. In addition to hands-on work in the clinic, I used computer skills to develop a system providing case management functions, electronic medical records using a SOAP format, prevention information, and accurate demographic data to serve as the basis for grant writing. Because the clinic operates at different sites across the county, the system is designed to be easily accessed anywhere while maintaining client confidentiality.

Experience Type: Paid Employment – Not Military
Most Meaningful Experience: No
Experience Name: Teaching Assistant, General Chemistry
Dates: 08/2009 – 05/2012
Hours/Week: 10
Experience Description: As a general chemistry teaching assistant, I prepared and taught a weekly general chemistry workshop to undergraduate and post-baccalaureate pre-medical students. I separately tutored small groups and individuals selected by the instructor as requiring the most assistance. Because many students doubted their abilities and often feared the material, I helped them build confidence and analytical skills through successful problem solving. I also ran popular comprehensive midterm and final review sessions.

Experience Type: Paid Employment – Not Military

Most Meaningful Experience: No
Experience Name: Private Tutor, General Physics
Dates: 05/2009 – 10/2010
Hours/Week: 6
Experience Description: After serving as a chemistry teaching assistant, several of my post-baccalaureate students asked me to privately tutor them in physics. I prepared practice exercises for our weekly meetings and carefully structured problem-solving exercises to match each student's current grasp of the material. It was quite satisfying to witness each student's improvement in both skill and confidence through the semester, with one student increasing her C grade to an A.

Experience Type: Research/Lab
Most Meaningful Experience: No
Experience Name: Research Assistant
Dates: 10/2008 – 12/2009
Hours/Week: 9
Experience Description: I worked at a laboratory studying the social function of emotions. As a research assistant, I coordinated data collection to examine shifts in self-understanding during experiences of compassion and pride. I collected EKG and skin conductance data from subjects exposed to emotionally powerful stimuli. I then wrote a program to rapidly aggregate physiological data, greatly improving the efficiency of a process formerly done by hand and allowing a more complete profile of subjects' emotional reactivity.

Experience Type: Paid Employment – Not Military
Most Meaningful Experience: No

Experience Name: Computer Programmer and Systems Analyst
Dates: 02/2003 – Present
Hours/Week: 20-40
Experience Description: While finishing my undergraduate degree and taking pre-medical courses, I have worked as a systems analyst and computer programmer in the information technology department of a nationally known 350-person law firm. I write programs to analyze business workflows, such as expense reimbursement. The job requires frequent interaction with and technical education of various constituencies including partners, junior attorneys, technical staff, secretaries, and software vendors. While in school, I was asked to serve as interim manager of a firm-wide upgrade to the desktop operating and document management systems. I write programs in C#, Java, JavaScript and VB.NET.

Experience Type: Community Service/Volunteer – Medical/ Clinical
Most Meaningful Experience: No
Experience Name: Preparing and Serving Food to People in Need
Dates: 01/2002 – 12/2003
Hours/Week: 5
Experience Description: I helped prepare, cook, and serve weekly meals at a "free restaurant" providing a hot meal to anyone who comes through the doors. I enjoyed the simple work of preparing meals because of the great respect offered to those who arrived to receive food. The atmosphere cultivated is not that of the more fortunate helping the less fortunate, but rather that of fellow human beings helping each other. My appreciation for this ethos led me to seek other organizations grounded in the ideal of a community caring for its own members.

Example 3: Padma's AMCAS Work/Activities

Padma's admissions elevator pitch:

First generation Sri Lankan who became interested in ophthalmology as a child requiring glasses and pursued interest through participating in free eye clinics for disadvantaged inner city populations, performing ophthalmology research, and founding sustainable eye clinic in Sri Lanka.

I rarely allow clients to include the maximum 15 work/activities. Padma is a rare exception to this rule. Notice how the vast majority of Padma's activities focus on her passion for ophthalmology, although these experiences fall into varying categories such as community service, research, and extracurricular activities. Use Padma's work/activities as a litmus test for how strong each activity needs to be if you decide to fill all 15 spaces.

Experience Type: Paid Employment – Not Military
Most Meaningful Experience: No
Experience Name: Clinical Research Coordinator
Dates: 10/2011 – Present
Hours/Week: 40
Experience Description: Motivated by a desire to gain greater clinical exposure, I currently work as a clinical research coordinator for a study examining the safety and effectiveness of a device used during glaucoma filtration surgery (trabeculectomy). I liaise between the sponsor and all eight sites and communicate daily with physicians, research coordinators, and regulatory personnel. Coordinating all data collection and analysis requires strong communication and

problem-solving skills. I have improved my ability to multi-task and manage competing demands between our site and other study sites. I enjoy interacting with patients, shadowing ophthalmologists weekly, and observing surgeries.

Experience Type: Honors/Awards/Recognitions
Most Meaningful Experience: No
Experience Name: Awards and Honors
Dates: 05/2011
Hours/Week:
Experience Description: In recognition of academic and extra-curricular achievements during my university career, I was named a finalist for the Rhodes Scholarship in May 2011. I was also placed on the Dean's List for the 2010-2011 academic year for achieving a GPA above 3.7 and received a Bachelor's of Arts in Biology magna cum laude for maintaining a cumulative GPA above 3.6 during my undergraduate career.

Experience Type: Honors/Awards/Recognitions
Most Meaningful Experience: No
Experience Name: Top 10 College Women
Dates: 09/2010
Hours/Week:
Experience Description: A leading US magazine named me one of the "Top 10 College Women." I was selected from college seniors across the US and Canada for this award valued at $5,000. Selection was based upon academic achievement, leadership experience, and involvement in community and campus affairs. Additionally, I was the recipient of the Beauty of Giving Award, chosen from among the "Top 10 College Women" award winners for

a $3,000 cash prize based on outstanding community service work.

Experience Type: Paid Employment – Not Military
Most Meaningful Experience: No
Experience Name: Research Intern
Dates: 05/2010 – 7/2010
Hours/Week: 40
Experience Description: I interned in the Health System Planning and Research Branch to understand how governmental health policies are informed and implemented. I worked on the "Externally-Informed Annual Health Systems Trends Report" exploring challenges to public health systems. I performed a literature search on health services research and identified relevant primary literature. Based on my performance, I wrote the section entitled, "Chronic Disease Prevention and Management," which critically evaluated more than 70 research articles. Overall, I became aware of the complexity of health care systems and the political, economic, and social contexts in which medicine is practiced.

Experience Type: Honors/Awards/Recognitions
Most Meaningful Experience: No
Experience Name: Named a "Young Leader of Social Change"
Dates: 04/2010
Hours/Week:
Experience Description: I received this award in both 2009 and 2010. I was recognized for work improving vision both locally and internationally, as well as for my independent projects with the Clinic for Diabetic Retinopathy (2009) and for my research project in Sri Lanka (2010). As a result, I was asked to speak at a global health innovation summit in 2009 and 2010.

Experience Type: Community Service/Volunteer – Medical/Clinical
Most Meaningful Experience: No
Experience Name: Peer Advisor
Dates: 09/2009 – 05/2011
Hours/Week: 1
Experience Description: I worked in conjunction with faculty, academic advisors, and house deans to help incoming freshmen transition to college life. I aided students in class selection and addressed non-academic concerns that arose during the summer before college. I enjoyed participating in New Student Orientation for incoming freshmen and remaining in contact with students throughout the academic year. As an advisor specifically for other University Scholars, I also helped students contact potential mentors for independent research. I am confident my ability to work collaboratively with numerous faculty members has prepared me well for a career in medicine that necessitates teamwork and cooperation.

Experience Type: Research/Lab
Most Meaningful Experience: Yes
Experience Name: Independent Research Project
Dates: 08/2009 – 8/2010
Hours/Week: 5
Experience Description: To augment my extracurricular work aimed at addressing avoidable blindness, I conducted research on childhood blindness in Bangladesh. I had read a paper reporting that girls in Bangladesh were significantly more likely than boys to suffer from preventable blindness. However, no reasons were provided for this finding. Thus, I proposed a research project to further examine the factors putting Bangladeshi girls at a greater risk of becoming blind due to preventable causes than boys. To answer this question, I sur-

veyed the primary caregivers of 88 blind children and 264 non-blind children in a case-controlled epidemiological study.

Most Meaningful Experience Remarks: This experience allowed me to apply skills and knowledge gained from biology, sociology, and statistics courses to a topic I was passionate about. In addition to proposing, organizing, and obtaining IRB approval for the study, I created a novel 50-item questionnaire to obtain information about family structure, education level, socio-economic status, and health beliefs, attitudes, and practices. I also conducted several field tests of the survey to ensure questions were culturally sensitive while remaining clinically relevant. Overall, I found the factors most predictive of childhood blindness in girls included mother's educational status, mother's comfort with seeking medical attention for her child, and the child's nutritional status. Although I worked under the guidance of professors from the US and England, neither was present during the data collection stage. As a result, the project required independence and self-directed learning. Living and working in the same villages as research subjects also required me to be versatile and adaptable, as I had to overcome any unexpected challenges on my own in an unfamiliar setting.

Experience Type: Extracurricular/Hobbies/Avocations
Most Meaningful Experience: Yes
Experience Name: Founder
Dates: 09/2008 – Present
Hours/Week: 4
Experience Description: In the summer of 2008, I read that the prevalence of diabetes in Sri Lanka was approximately ten times the global level. At the time, only one clinic in the capital city of Colombo was capable of carrying out tests needed for a comprehensive

diagnosis of diabetic retinopathy, a common complication of diabetes. Yet, the tests costs were prohibitively expensive for the average Sri Lankan. Over the course of the next year, I performed research to draft a proposal for a clinic that would provide free vision screenings and follow-up for diabetic retinopathy according to standards set forth by the World Health Organization's Vision 2020 Initiative.

Most Meaningful Experience Remarks: My involvement represented a sustained commitment to helping solve a problem others had previously recognized but never acted on. I spent several months in Sri Lanka between 2008 and 2009 to help establish the clinic and have traveled back to visit the clinic every few months. I gained a solid understanding of the state of vision care in Sri Lanka, and then designed a proposal for the clinic based on what I had observed as strengths and weaknesses of the current system. Through this project, I became familiar with medical terminology relating to this area of medicine as I read textbooks and clinical guidelines to understand international standards for care of diabetic retinopathy. This experience demanded professionalism and strong communication skills as I collaborated with physicians, hospital administrators, representatives from the Sri Lankan Ministry of Healthcare and Nutrition, and potential funding partners. I persistently presented my plan for the clinic both confidently and knowledgeably to articulate why exactly this model, proposed by a young student raised abroad, provided a novel method for addressing a growing problem in Sri Lanka. The clinic now screens and provides follow-up care for hundreds of patients each month.

Experience Type: Research/Lab
Most Meaningful Experience: Yes
Experience Name: Research Assistant

Dates: 09/2008 – 9/2011

Hours/Week: 10

Experience Description: I helped design research protocols and tested animal subjects to explore the potential for gene therapy in patients with inherited eye diseases causing severe visual impairment and blindness. I worked alongside other lab members on projects utilizing techniques such as cryosectioning, microscopy, retinal dissection, perfusion, and testing of the optokinetic nystagmus reflex (OKR). This early commitment to the lab gave me the background and confidence needed to pose my own scientific questions. For my senior thesis, I investigated how the retinal anatomy of the CEP290-/- mouse (a model for Leber's Congenital Amaurosis in humans) changes during the postnatal weeks 1-6.

Most Meaningful Experience Remarks: This experience allowed me to gain a deeper understanding of the process of translational research. I used microscopy, pupillometry, and a test of the OKR to find that CEP290-/- mice are born with photoreceptor cells, but these cells degenerate with time and cause the retina to thin. The inner and outer segments, the outer nuclear layer, and the outer plexiform layer are particularly vulnerable to degeneration. This data can then be used as a baseline against which to measure the effectiveness of proposed gene therapy treatments. Working in basic research challenged me to be diligent, patient, and persistent. Additionally, the lab introduced me to the potential end results of successful translational research. The principal investigator was treating 12 LCA patients in a clinical trial using AAV injection, and I helped analyze the study data. It was extremely rewarding to observe the patients' marked improvement in vision and quality of life following the treatment. This remarkable experience has inspired me to remain committed to translational research throughout my future career in medicine.

Experience Type: Research/Lab
Most Meaningful Experience: No
Experience Name: Research Assistant
Dates: 09/2008 – 5/2010
Hours/Week: 4

Experience Description: Over the course of two years, I became familiar with all stages of research study design, implementation, and reporting. I worked on a study examining the influence of nurse staffing on patient outcomes in the Neonatal Intensive Care Unit. I helped recruit hospitals, amend the survey, and manage a database of 104 hospitals and more than 5,000 nurses. I also used statistical packages such as SPSS to make regression models and other data analyses. I prepared initial drafts of manuscripts and assisted in writing NIH grants for the center. The experience reinforced the need for collaboration and teamwork in patient care and the invaluable role of nurses in improving patient outcomes.

Experience Type: Community Service/Volunteer – Medical/Clinical
Most Meaningful Experience: No
Experience Name: Global Impact Corps Volunteer
Dates: 06/2008 – 07/2008
Hours/Week: 30

Experience Description: I worked alongside ophthalmologists, optometrists, and other volunteers based at an eye clinic in Chennai, India. I learned how to test a patient's visual acuity and use a slit lamp. We traveled to villages, slums, and schools to provide free vision screenings to low-income individuals. I observed cataract surgeries and regularly shadowed doctors. Additionally, I participated in outreach programs to teach individuals about good health practices needed to protect one's vision. From this hands-on experience, I gained appreciation for an integrated approach to patient care, which incorporates research evidence, public health initiatives, and direct patient care.

Experience Type: Extracurricular/Hobbies/Avocations
Most Meaningful Experience: No
Experience Name: Pilates
Dates: 09/2007 – Present
Hours/Week: 1
Experience Description: During my college career, I enjoyed participating in Pilates group classes as a way of unwinding in a healthy and productive manner. I took reformer and matte Pilates classes both at my university and a private studio. Pilates is based on precise, controlled movements requiring steady concentration. I found it rewarding to see gradual changes in my body resulting from consistent dedication to the Pilates methods. I eventually sought to introduce others to my love of Pilates and completed training to become a Pilates Method Alliance-certified beginner matte instructor in October 2010.

Experience Type: Community Service/Volunteer – Medical/Clinical
Most Meaningful Experience: No
Experience Name: Volunteer and Board Member
Dates: 09/2006 – 05/2010
Hours/Week: 2
Experience Description: For all four years of college, I served as a volunteer with my university's chapter of a volunteer organization dedicated to improving the vision of all. As the chair of vision screenings, I organized and conducted vision screenings at soup kitchens and schools in the inner city. I also assisted with leading community health fairs that provided education on eye health and referrals to free

vision care. Additionally, as vice president, I helped the chapter secure increased funding from the university. I was named Chapter Volunteer of the Year in 2008 when I helped raise over $1,500 for international programs.

Experience Type: Teaching/Tutoring
Most Meaningful Experience: No
Experience Name: Elementary School Tutor
Dates: 09/2007 – 5/2008
Hours/Week: 2
Experience Description: I volunteered at an elementary school in the inner city. Each week, I tutored and mentored second grade students performing below grade level in math and English. I improved communication skills as I catered to each student's needs and creatively devised reinforcement activities drawing upon the student's personal interests to make the coursework more relevant. I also completed cultural sensitivity training to gain a better understanding of the diverse demographic and socioeconomic traits of the students. I enjoyed tangibly measuring the students' progress over the year through improved test scores and reading abilities.

Experience Type: Honors/Awards/Recognitions
Most Meaningful Experience: No
Experience Name: University Scholars Scholarship
Dates: 09/2006
Hours/Week:
Experience Description: I was one of twenty-five freshmen students from an incoming class of over 2,500 awarded this research scholarship. I was selected based on my high school research pursuits and expressed interest in pursuing independent research projects

in university. The scholarship included funding for all research activities (I secured a $3,000 grant to fund research in Bangladesh), mentorship from distinguished professors, and access to honors coursework. My involvement with the University Scholars program culminated in an oral presentation of my research results from Bangladesh in March 2010.

Example 4: Mary's AMCAS Work/Activities

Mary's admissions elevator pitch:

> *MD/PhD candidate whose interest in research started while teaching music to autistic child and who used patience, thoughtful reflection, and communication skills practiced as singer to advance scientific investigations.*

Given Mary is applying MD/PhD, her AMCAS work/activities section is expectedly research heavy. But look how she incorporates other activities such as volunteering, tutoring, and singing to highlight qualities that will make her an outstanding physician in addition to a leading researcher. Also observe how she groups similar activities under one theme (undergraduate research presentations, graduate research presentations, undergraduate awards, graduate awards, *etc.*) to make the work/activities section easier to read. Please note Mary initially included full, formal research citations, but these have been edited to maintain her anonymity.

Experience Type: Publications
Most Meaningful Experience: No
Experience Name: Publications

Dates: 01/2012
Hours/Week:
Experience Description: 1. Glucose Dynamics in Ovarian Follicles. (2012). Bird et al. *Molecule and Cell.* 450(1):493-96. 2. Vascular Injuries After Knee Replacement. (2009). Schenecker et al. *Arthroplasty.* (25):1345-47. 3. Knee Replacement Complications. (2009). Schenecker et al. *Arthroplasty.* (28):1748-51.

Experience Type: Community Service/Volunteer – Medical/Clinical
Most Meaningful Experience: Yes
Experience Name: Autism Buddies, Big Buddy Volunteer
Dates: 09/2011 – Until Present
Hours/Week: 4
Experience Description: Serve as a playmate and mentor for seven-year-old girl with autism to help her strengthen communication and socialization skills.
Most Meaningful Experience Remarks: "I might not remember your name or where you're from, but I will remember that your work could help my baby someday." These were the words of Sally's mother when she learned I work in a neurobiology lab at NIH. Even though I am not directly studying autism, Sally's mother believes neuronal gene expression investigations could be applicable in helping her daughter. Her words filled me with a sense of responsibility and purpose. Interacting with Sally and her mother continually reminds me people are the ultimate purpose for biomedical research and research provides solutions and hope. At the same time, this experience helped me conclusively decide I must work with patients in my career. I felt great satisfaction watching Sally make noticeable progress during our time together. At our first session, she seemed distant, detached, and uninterested in social

interaction. After several months, she greeted me with a hug and a smile and would not leave my side. The most humbling and fulfilling day was when Sally finally sang the words to a song I had been teaching her all year. By remaining patient and consistent, I helped Sally approach ordinary tasks from new angles, and I learned how meaningful directly helping others can be.

Experience Type: Research/Lab
Most Meaningful Experience: Yes
Experience Name: Research Training Award
Dates: 06/2011 – Until Present
Hours/Week: 40
Experience Description: As a Technical Intramural Research Training Award Fellow at NIH, I study gene expression in rat neurons with a focus on local translation in axons of superior cervical ganglia (SCG) primary neurons. I dissect SCGs and maintain the compartmentalized culture system for the lab, design and execute experiments independently, and present experimental data at weekly lab meetings. I also discuss interpretations of results with the postdocs, lab manager, and principal investigator and attend relevant lectures, courses, and journal clubs. I am first author of a manuscript currently in preparation.
Most Meaningful Experience Remarks: After college, I wanted to conduct research at NIH more than anything. I applied for an NIH Post-baccalaureate Intramural Research Training Award (IRTA) but did not land a position. Determined to get to NIH, I reapplied following my masters, this time for a Technical IRTA. With persistence and focus, I reached my goal. Working at NIH is a continual source of inspiration for pursuing science. In addition to improving technical and critical thinking skills, I have learned

communicating science is as important as performing it and am eager to disseminate basic science knowledge to clinical practitioners during my career. I thrive in this competitive and stimulating biomedical research environment where I have the privilege of hearing prominent scientists discuss research findings at weekly lectures and of shadowing monthly in the ICU. This research and clinical combination provides the exciting balance I hope to maintain through a career in translational research.

Experience Type: Presentations/Posters
Most Meaningful Experience: No
Experience Name: Poster Presentations of Master's Research
Dates: 10/2010
Hours/Week:
Experience Description: 1. Nql4p Telomere Maintenance. Lee at al. Cell Biology Conference, San Francisco, CA (10/10). 2. Telomere RNA Processing Proteins. Lee et al. Xi Symposium, NYU (4/10). 3. Post-transcriptional Regulation of Gene Expression. Raferty et al. European Network, Bilbao, Spain (10/09). 4. Telomere RNA Processing Proteins. Raferty et al. College Research Symposium. (7/09). 5. Regulating Telomere Length. Raferty and Lee. Xi Symposium, NYU (4/09).

Experience Type: Presentations/Posters
Most Meaningful Experience: No
Experience Name: Poster Presentations of Undergraduate Research
Dates: 07/2009
Hours/Week:
Experience Description: 1. Luteinization of Granulosa Cells. Macon et al. Reproduction Annual Meeting, Orlando, FL. (7/09).

2. Luteinization of Granulosa Cells. Raferty et al. Annual Student Research and Scholarship Colloquium. Baltimore, MD (4/08). Recipient of 3rd Place Award for best poster of Mathematics and Natural Sciences Posters.

Experience Type: Teaching/Tutoring
Most Meaningful Experience: No
Experience Name: Teaching Assistant
Dates: 07/2009 – 06/2010
Hours/Week: 15
Experience Description: 1. Selected as teaching assistant for the Howard Hughes Medical Institute college research course. In this yearlong intensive course, students isolate bacteriophages from the soil and annotate genomes of novel phages for publication. 2. Annotated novel genome "Bluebird" now in GenBank. Assisted students with laboratory procedures, encouraged scientific inquiry, and communicated excitement for research. 3. State Teaching Assistantship for undergrad biology labs: Cells, Comparative Anatomy, Genetics, & Developmental Biology (9/08-6/10).

Experience Type: Research/Lab
Most Meaningful Experience: No
Experience Name: Masters Thesis Research
Dates: 10/2009 – 06/2011
Hours/Week: 30
Experience Description: Studied telomere biology with a focus on the involvement of yeast RNA processing proteins in the protection of telomeres while mentoring and training undergraduate research students and summer scholars. Presented research at

numerous conferences and received funding from biology department to present research at an international conference in Spain. Improved technical and analytical skills and gained a great appreciation for research. The investigation culminated in a written thesis and public defense seminar given during the State Biology Department Seminar Series (6/11).

Experience Type: Honors/Awards/Recognitions
Most Meaningful Experience: No
Experience Name: Masters Degree Academic Honors and Awards
Dates: 05/2009
Hours/Week:
Experience Description: 1. Graduate Biology Merit Award for class of 2011 top biology scholar (5/11). 2. National Honor Society for graduate and professional students (5/11-present). 3. Higher Education Travel Grant Award to attend Translational Research Symposium & MD/PhD Career Development Workshop, Houston, TX (1/11). 4. Scientific Research Society (5/09-present). 5. Graduate Assistantship with full tuition scholarship and stipend for masters in Biology (9/09-6/11).

Experience Type: Honors/Awards/Recognitions
Most Meaningful Experience: No
Experience Name: Undergraduate Academic Honors and Awards
Dates: 05/2009
Hours/Week:
Experience Description: 1. Selected to sing national anthem at 2008 commencement ceremony (5/09). 2. Cum Laude Honors at graduation (5/09). 3. National Biological Honor Society (4/09-present). 4. Music department vocal scholarship (12/07) (Contact Jeremy

Anderson, anderson@marylandstate.edu). 5. Dean's List honors during five semesters (Fall06, Fall07, Spring08, Fall08, Spring09). 6. Four-year Tuition Exchange Scholarship (9/05).

Experience Type: Research/Lab
Most Meaningful Experience: No
Experience Name: Undergraduate Research
Dates: 01/2009 – 06/2009
Hours/Week: 15
Experience Description: Investigated roles of glucose and metabolites in luteinization of granulosa cells in the Rhesus macaque ovary. Presented posters at several conferences. Gave a research seminar entitled, "Luteinization of Granulosa Cells," as an invited speaker for the Biological Honor Society Seminar Series (2/09). Authored a publication in *Molecule and Cell* (1/12).

Experience Type: Leadership – not Listed Elsewhere
Most Meaningful Experience: Yes
Experience Name: Musical director of *a cappella* group
Dates: 09/2007 – 05/2009
Hours/Week: 15
Experience Description: Sang in all-female *a cappella* group for four years of college and was elected musical director during junior and senior years. Arranged songs, taught vocal parts, ran rehearsals, and conducted performances. Led group to participate in first off-campus *a cappella* festival and encouraged application for a performance spot in the International Collegiate Championship of *a cappella* (ICCA). Designed the ICCA set list and organized our first appearance in ICCAs. Learned how to unite a diverse group of people to pursue a common goal.

Most Meaningful Experience Remarks: From the moment I was accepted as a freshman, I aspired to become the group's musical director and achieved this goal junior year. When I began as director, morale was low. However, I knew we had the potential to make great music if we worked hard. Therefore, I increased the number of practices from two to three per week, expanded our audience by performing in the community, and continuously provided positive reinforcement. By the end of my initial year as director, we entered our first ICCA competition and won third place, best soloist, and best vocal percussion. Through hard work and devotion, I led the group to a higher level, and the group continues to maintain this standard. Beyond the musical challenges of songwriting and conducting, this position taught me how to unite people of differing personality types, mediate conflicts, and mentor prospective leaders. As director, I cultivated strong leadership skills that I look forward to using as a physician.

Experience Type: Other
Most Meaningful Experience: No
Experience Name: Clinically/Medically Relevant Experiences
Dates: 06/2007 – Until Present
Hours/Week:
Experience Description: 1. ICU Rounds Shadowing Program at NIH, 9/11-present, monthly. Contact shadowingprogram@gmail.com. 2. President of American Medical Student Association, 6/11-5/12. Attended 2011 National Convention. Contact Rod Lambert, 301-555-2594. 3. Shadowed Dr. Geraldine Masters, general surgeon, Community Hospital, 10/08. Contact Dr. Geraldine Masters, 301.555.2356. 4. Shadowed Dr. Meha Lambozi, orthopedic surgeon, Philadelphia Hospital, summers 07/08. Contact Meha Lam-

bozi, 215.555.7823. 5. Shadowed Dr. John Purdy, orthopedic surgeon, Philadelphia Hospital, 7/08. Contact Jonathan Purdy, 215.555.7825.

Experience Type: Research/Lab
Most Meaningful Experience: No
Experience Name: Clinical Research
Dates: 05/2007 – 08/2008
Hours/Week: 40
Experience Description: Completed two, 10-week summer internships as a student researcher in bone and joint research (summers 2007, 2008). Interviewed postoperative patients to assess pain and activity levels. Managed and organized patient data for a six-year prospective study assessing local and systemic in-hospital complications following total hip/knee replacements. Authored two publications in *Arthroplasty*. Presented this research as an invited speaker for Biology Department Seminar Series, 10/07.

Experience Type: Community Service/Volunteer – Medical/Clinical
Most Meaningful Experience: No
Experience Name: Hospital Volunteer Experiences
Dates: 06/2006 – 05/2009
Hours/Week: 3
Experience Description: 1. Volunteered in Center for Neonatal Transitional Care at Washington Pediatric Hospital (10/08-5/09, 2hr/wk). Held and rocked pre-mature, developmentally delayed, and drug addicted infants. Helped infants and toddlers attain specific developmental goals through stimulation with rehabilitation toys. 2. Premed Volunteer at Pennsylvania Hospital (6/06-8/06, 4hr/wk). Volunteered on inpatient surgical unit and transported

patients to x-rays/diagnostic tests. Tended to patients needs by bringing water and bedding.

Experience Type: Community Service/Volunteer – not Medical/ Clinical
Most Meaningful Experience: No
Experience Name: Food Pantry and Community Center Volunteer Experiences
Dates: 09/2010 – 03/2011
Hours/Week:
Experience Description: 1. Served hot meals to needy community members at the Community Center in Philadelphia, PA (6/10-3/11, monthly) 2. Packaged food at Food Pantry and Emergency Financial Assistance Center in Baltimore, MD (9/03/12/04, 2hr/ wk). Played games with children when their families visited center. Designed handmade greeting cards for "CARDS for CARES" fundraising project.

Example 5: Gabbi's AMCAS Work/Activities

Gabbi's admissions elevator pitch:

African-American woman who attended traditionally black college, served in sorority and club leadership roles, worked in free clinic serving indigent minority patients, and wants to become primary care physician focusing on decreasing health disparities in black communities.

Gabbi, though applying during the summer of junior year in order to head directly to medical school, does an excellent job of using the work/activities section to highlight leadership experience and desire to reduce health disparities in African American communities. She presents these ideas through her work/activities, and then fleshes them out more fully in the personal statement (which you will find in the Essays Section). Also note how she doesn't shy away from sorority experiences and presents her time in "Greek" life in a convincingly positive manner.

Experience Type: Honors/Awards/Recognitions
Most Meaningful Experience: No
Experience Name: Hill Scholarship
Dates: 09/2011 – 6/2012
Hours/Week:
Experience Description: The Hill Scholarship of $1000 is awarded to a member of Alpha Sorority. I received the award because of my service and leadership within the sorority and my superior representation of the sorority through academics, leadership, and community service.

Experience Type: Research/Lab
Most Meaningful Experience: No
Experience Name: "Cardiac Components of Anxiety"
Dates: 1/2011 – Until Present
Hours/Week: 10
Experience Description: In this study, we introduce test subjects to tasks that measure parasympathetic functioning (attention via stroop task) and sympathetic functioning (flight/fight via math task) while recording heart rate variability. Heart rate variability is believed to provide a measure of an individual's autonomic space. We also compare self-reported behavioral responses to anxiety driv-

en situations with the goal of determining where participants lie in autonomic space and how this relates to self-reporting. I have learned how to effectively place electrodes on participants and how to "clean" data. I have also enjoyed working one-on-one with participants.

Experience Type: Honors/Awards/Recognitions
Most Meaningful Experience: No
Experience Name: Who's Who
Dates: 11/2010
Hours/Week:
Experience Description: Who's Who Among Students in American Colleges and Universities is a national program recognizing college students for outstanding leadership, scholarship, and service. Each fall outstanding students nominated by college faculty and staff submit applications for this recognition opportunity.

Experience Type: Other
Most Meaningful Experience: No
Experience Name: Clinical Experience
Dates: 10/2010 – 02/2011
Hours/Week:
Experience Description: On various occasions, I have spent free time gaining clinical experience at University Hospital by shadowing Dr. Frank Davidson in emergency medicine and Dr. Mitch Yervis in pediatrics. While shadowing Dr. Davidson, I saw the examination and treatment of a diverse set of chief complaints, from painful vaginal bleeding to diabetic ketoacidosis. While shadowing Dr. Yervis, I observed newborn exams and treatment for premature birth complications.

Experience Type: Community Service/Volunteer – not Medical/Clinical
Most Meaningful Experience: No
Experience Name: Co-mentor
Dates: 09/2010 – Until Present
Hours/Week:
Experience Description: My mentor informed me of an opportunity to help a young woman named Ayesha who lives in a group home because of family issues. Ayesha hoped to attend college but needed assistance with studying for the SAT. I provided one-on-one SAT tutoring and developed a home study plan. We also discussed her ultimate goal of becoming a psychologist. She was recently accepted into DC College's bridge program, which, upon completion, will allow her to attend a four-year university.

Experience Type: Paid Employment – not Military
Most Meaningful Experience: Yes
Experience Name: Resident Assistant/Office Conference Assistant
Dates: 08/2010 – Until Present
Hours/Week: 40
Experience Description: As a resident assistant during the school year, I mentor freshman residents and ensure enforcement of dormitory policies. I also assist students with roommate concerns, school issues, and conflict resolution. As an office conference assistant during the summer, I help the residence hall community director prepare for incoming summer residents. I also greet new summer residents and help check them into the building.
Most Meaningful Experience Remarks: My time as a resident assistant has provided invaluable skills as a leader and mentor. I was initially intimidated by the position due to stories circulated about

the tenuous conflicts I would be responsible for handling among the forty residents under my charge. However, once the school year started, and I developed relationships with each resident, I learned to love the position. I made clear the kind of behavior I expected from them, and conflict on the floor was a non-issue. The residents not only respected me as their authority figure, but also trusted me as a friend, and would come to me with rooming issues, school difficulties, and relationship problems. When I learned a portion of my residents struggled academically during their first semester, I started study halls to help them improve. Similarly, I planned a sexual health program to educate the residents when I learned of a pregnancy and case of herpes on our floor. I so enjoyed my time as resident assistant that I will continue the position during the next school year.

Experience Type: Other
Most Meaningful Experience: Yes
Experience Name: Summer Medical and Dental Educational Program (SMDEP)
Dates: 06/2010 – 07/2010
Hours/Week: 45
Experience Description: During the Summer Medical and Dental Educational Program, I took condensed courses on genetics, biochemistry, HIPAA policy, healthcare ethics, health policy, and health disparities. I also gained clinical experience shadowing doctors in the University Hospital pediatric and family medicine departments. In addition, I made lifelong friends who share similar medical goals.
Most Meaningful Experience Remarks: The Summer Medical and Dental Educational program solidified my desire to become a physician. A lecture on health disparities revealed the disappointing

health disparities affecting those of my race – African Americans. For example, HIV/AIDS, diabetes, heart disease, stroke, and even cancer seem to affect my race more than others. I also learned about the reasons for these disparities, which include high-stress environments, lack of access to and poor quality of care, and minimal representation in the health care field. After this lecture, it became clear I had a personal responsibility to become a physician in order to help reduce the disparities in my community.

Experience Type: Leadership – not Listed Elsewhere
Most Meaningful Experience: Yes
Experience Name: Leadership and membership Alpha Sorority
Dates: 03/2010 – Until Present
Hours/Week: 45
Experience Description: I have been an active member of Alpha Sorority since induction in the spring of 2010 by attending the majority of chapter meetings, programs, and community service events. In the summer of 2010, I was appointed to be the chapter's corresponding secretary and ran all communication between members while continuously updating the chapter's calendar of events. I was recently elected to be chapter treasurer for this coming school year. In addition, I was appointed to be a chairwoman for this year's Alpha week, a week dedicated to the sorority's initiatives.
Most Meaningful Experience Remarks: Being initiated into Alpha Sorority introduced me to a wonderful sisterhood while enhancing my confidence and determination to live up to the "Alpha Excellent" example placed before me. Before Alpha, I struggled with confidence issues. However, when I became a member of this prestigious sorority, I had no choice but to hold myself above the highest standards. So, with the encouragement of my "big sisters," I

summoned the courage to become vice president of the College of Arts and Sciences Honors Association, a resident assistant at a freshman dormitory, and corresponding secretary of Alpha, all during my junior year. Because of my success in each of these positions, I will continue to develop leadership skills during my senior year.

Experience Type: Leadership – not Listed Elsewhere
Most Meaningful Experience: No
Experience Name: Leadership and membership in College of Arts and Sciences Honors Association (CASHA)
Dates: 08/2009 – Until Present
Hours/Week:
Experience Description: I have been an active member of the College of Arts and Sciences Honors Association (CASHA) since my induction as a sophomore. My first year in CASHA, I attended a majority of the general body meetings and community service events. My second year, I was elected vice president and helped organize CASHA meetings and events. I also planned a time management program, where members of CASHA advised freshman how to schedule study time and provided study tips. I was recently elected president of CASHA and will start the position this coming school year.

Experience Type: Community Service/Volunteer – not Medical/Clinical
Most Meaningful Experience: No
Experience Name: Volunteering at Washington Pediatric Hospital
Dates: 06/2009 – 08/2009
Hours/Week: 6
Experience Description: During my time volunteering at Washing-

ton Pediatric Hospital, I provided patients with recreational activities between medical procedures and assisted with administrative duties. I also shadowed Dr. Baily Lovette as she carried out her daily routine of examining and treating patients and during meetings with parents and guardians.

Experience Type: Honors/Awards/Recognitions
Most Meaningful Experience: No
Experience Name: Chemistry Department's Chemical Rubber Company Award
Dates: 04/2009
Hours/Week:
Experience Description: I earned the Chemistry Department's Chemical Rubber Company Award because of my outstanding performance in General Chemistry I. Not only did I frequently receive the highest grades in the class on tests, but I also helped set up study sessions for classmates who had difficulty with the class material.

Experience Type: Other
Most Meaningful Experience: No
Experience Name: Academic Awards
Dates: 08/2008 – Until Present
Hours/Week:
Experience Description:
1. Legacy Scholarship, 2008 – present: covers full tuition and fees.
2. Dean's List of the College of Arts and Sciences, 2008 – present.
3. Quadrangle Honors, 2009 and 2011: for academic success while living in the dorm. 4. Alpha Sorority's 4.0 Club, 2011: for attaining a 4.0 GPA while in the sorority. 5. Parker Academic Award,

2011: $500 funded by Educational Foundation for having highest GPA in Alpha Sorority's chapter.

Experience Type: Extracurricular/Hobbies/Avocations
Most Meaningful Experience: No
Experience Name: Campus Societies' Memberships
Dates: 08/2008 – Until Present
Hours/Week:
Experience Description: I am a member of the following societies on my university's campus: 1.The Health Professions Society exposes pre-professional students to activities and opportunities that will help them become competitive candidates for Health Professions Schools. 2. National Society of Scholars is an honor society that invites high-achieving (top 20% of class) college students and provides resources for its members. 3. Scientific Honor Society encourages and advances scientific educations and invites high achievers in those areas. 4. International Honor Society is an academic honor society that recognizes and encourages scholastic achievement and excellence.

AMCAS Section VI: Letters of Evaluation

AMCAS refers to recommendations as "letters of evaluation." These recommendations are another chance for you to shape your medical school application story and show well roundedness. Most schools require at least three recommendations and often want two of them to be written by science professors. I suggest obtaining at least five letters of evaluation and sending them all if the school allows it, and if you are confident all the recommendations are strong. If a school has a maximum of three letters of evaluation, choose the three you believe will be best received by that specific school.

AMCAS allows you to designate which recommendations are sent to each school. Varying the recommendation letters sent is common practice because each school has its own evaluation letter rules. AMCAS allows you to enter up to 10 recommendations, but please do not send 10 letters to any one school. It is always better to send fewer strong recommendations than more mediocre ones. It only takes one lukewarm letter to tarnish an application.

Many undergraduate institutions provide a pre-med committee or advisor letter. These letters fall into three categories:

1. Pre-Med Committee Composite Letter – Pre-med committee writes a letter composed of excerpts from the letters you already obtained. This is often the only letter sent.
2. Pre-Med Committee Advisor Letter – A unique letter written by the pre-med advisor sent along with your other full letters.
3. Letter Packet – The school pre-med committee takes responsibility for sending each full letter you have obtained in one packet. The committee does not write a unique letter.

Ask your school's pre-med committee if it provides such a letter, how you go about obtaining one, and where your recommenders should send their letters. In general, if your school provides a pre-med committee letter, the medical school admissions committees want to see the letter regardless of your undergraduate course of study. Even if you are many years out of college or do not have a good relationship with your advisor, applying without a committee letter from a school that provides one is a red flag for admissions committees.

Though AMCAS does not start accepting letters of evaluation before May 1 of the application year, you should ask recommenders for letters when they will best remember you. This is often right after you complete a class or activity. You may ask the recommenders to write the letter and hold it on their computers until you apply. They can easily update the letter just prior to your application.

How can recommendation letters, given their content is written and controlled by the author, shape your application story? By strategically picking recommenders and instructing each on the letter's focus. It is acceptable to give each recommender the points you hope will be highlighted in the letter. Let's follow our pre-meds Tyler, Kevin, Padma, Mary, and Gabbi and see how they picked recommenders to further their story and asked for three points to be emphasized in each letter.

TYLER

Junior in large public university inspired by grandfather's 40-year career as family practitioner who confirmed importance of medicine's personal side through serving as EMT, Big Brother, and clinical research assistant.

Tyler uses a smart technique to obtain two science professor letters, while still allowing room for recommendations from his Big Brother director, EMT supervisor, and lacrosse coach. He asks the research supervisor, who also happens to be a professor and physician, to write the second "science letter."

Recommender	Letter Focus
Science professor	Academic prowess
	Analytical skills
	Intellect
Research supervisor/	Problem solving ability
Professor/	Teamwork
Orthopedist	Interest in surgery
Big Brother Director	Mentoring skills
	Compassion for less fortunate
	Affable personality
EMT Supervisor	Ease with patients
	Interest in clinical medicine
	Ability to work under pressure
Lacrosse Coach	Leadership
	Determination
	Teamwork

KEVIN

Forty-year-old software developer returned to pre-med post-baccalaureate courses after caring for friends dying of AIDS and subsequently worked as HIV counselor, developed software for free clinic, and performed psychiatric research. He hopes to become internist or psychiatrist working with patients suffering from chronic disease.

Kevin is a non-traditional candidate who needs to emphasize academic excellence while highlighting remarkable research and clinical experiences. He accomplishes this task by choosing five evaluators: two science professors, a research supervisor, and two clinical supervisors.

Recommender	Letter Focus
Science professor	Academic prowess
	Analytical skills
	Intellect
Second Science Professor	Reconfirm academic prowess
	Determination
	Cooperative approach to academics
Research supervisor	Problem solving skills
	Ability to apply IT knowledge to research
	Teamwork skills
HIV Counselor Supervisor	Trust building with patients
	Compassion
	Commitment
Free Clinic Supervisor	Dedication to underserved
	Bedside manner
	Initiative to create electronic records

PADMA

First generation Sri Lankan who became interested in oph-thalmology as a child requiring glasses and pursued interest through participating in free eye clinics for disadvantaged inner city populations, performing ophthalmology research, and founding sustainable eye clinic in Sri Lanka.

Padma follows what is often the best strategy for choosing recommenders – one science professor, second science professor with research focus, humanities professor, community service supervisor, and clinical experience supervisor. Padma emphasizes her passion for ophthalmology while still appearing well rounded.

Recommender	Letter Focus
Science professor	Academic prowess
	Analytical skills
	Intellect
Research supervisor/	Problem solving skills
Ophthalmologist	Teamwork skills
	Interest in ophthalmology
Humanities professor	Writing ability
	Public speaking talent
	Personal skills
Free eye clinics supervisor	Commitment
	Ease with patients
	Contagious energy
Physician from	Leadership skills
Sri Lankan Clinic	Compassion for poor
	Determination

MARY

MD/PhD candidate whose interest in research started while teaching music to autistic child and who used patience, thoughtful reflection, and communication skills practiced as singer to advance scientific investigations.

Mary, as an MD/PhD candidate, chooses six letters because she needs to emphasize research experiences while still showing well roundedness. Notice how she uses her music teacher as an evaluator.

Recommender	Letter Focus
Science professor	Academic prowess
	Analytical skills
	Intellect
Research supervisor/ NIH	Technical research skills
	Problem-solving skills
	Motivation
Research Supervisor/ Masters	Natural proclivity for research
	Determination
	Ingenuity
Research Supervisor/ Undergraduate	Inquisitive
	Hard worker
	Reliable
Big Buddy Supervisor	Commitment
	Ease with autistic child
	Compassion
Music Teacher	Creativity
	Resolve
	Artistic talent

GABBI

African-American woman who attended traditionally black college, served in sorority and club leadership roles, worked in free clinic serving indigent minority patients, and wants to become primary care physician focusing on decreasing health disparities in black communities.

Gabby decides to skip the humanities professor and clinical recommendations to include two science professors and a research supervisor. But she smartly uses a science professor who can comment on her desire to solve health disparities. Further, she highlights leadership skills in sorority and resident assistant supervisor recommendations.

Recommender	Letter Focus
Science professor	Academic prowess
	Analytical skills
	Intellect
Second science professor/ Mentor	Aptitude with complex concepts
	Hard worker
	desire to solve health disparities
Research Supervisor	Inquisitive
	Dedicated
	Problem-solving skills
Sorority Supervisor	Leadership skills
	Commitment
	Passion for serving others
Resident Assistant Supervisor	Leadership skills
	Conflict resolution skills
	Engaging personality

How do you let the recommenders know what qualities to highlight in the evaluation letter? You tell them. Set up an in-person meeting and ask the recommender directly if he or she can provide a strong recommendation. If the answer is an unabashed "yes!" then hand the recommender:

1. Updated resume
2. Transcript copies
3. Personal statement (if complete)
4. Recommendation deadline (make it three weeks before published deadline)
5. *Three items you want the recommender to highlight*
6. How to submit the recommendation by providing material such as the AMCAS Letter Request Form or your undergraduate pre-med committee address

Remember to waive your right to see the recommendation and be sure to write a thank you note to each recommender.

This book provides an overview of the medical school admissions process so you can begin preparing for it now. Detailed information about asking for recommendations, the specifics of recommendation services, and examples of "thank you" notes are available in my companion book, *The Medical School Admissions Guide*.

AMCAS Section VII: Medical Schools

The Medical Schools Section allows you to list where you want to apply. First, you need to know what schools are available to you. Here is a list of allopathic (MD) and osteopathic (DO) medical schools in the US by state based on data from the AAMC and

Wikipedia websites. You will notice many new schools have been founded in the last decade. Be sure to check if any new schools have been started before you apply, as they may be less competitive initially. And remember DO schools and Texas state regular MD schools have their own application services separate from AMCAS.

UNITED STATES MEDICAL SCHOOLS

State	Name	Degree	First Class
Alabama	University of Alabama School of Medicine	MD	1860
Alabama	University of South Alabama	MD	1972
Alabama	Alabama College of Osteopathic Medicine	DO	2013
Arizona	University of Arizona College of Medicine	MD	1967
Arizona	A.T. Still University School of Osteopathic Medicine in Arizona	DO	2011
Arizona	Midwestern University Arizona College of Osteopathic Medicine	DO	2000
Arkansas	University of Arkansas College of Medicine	MD	1880
California	David Geffen School of Medicine at UCLA	MD	1951
California	Keck School of Medicine of the University of Southern California	MD	1888
California	Loma Linda University School of Medicine	MD	1914
California	Stanford University School of Medicine	MD	1913

California	UCLA/Drew Medical Education Program	MD	1978
California	University of California – Davis School of Medicine	MD	1966
California	University of California – Irvine College of Medicine	MD	1896
California	University of California – Riverside School of Medicine	MD	2013
California	University of California – San Diego School of Medicine	MD	1968
California	University of California – San Francisco School of Medicine	MD	1973
California	Touro University California College of Osteopathic Medicine	DO	2001
California	Western University of Health Science	DO	1982
Colorado	University of Colorado Health Sciences Center School of Medicine	MD	1885
Colorado	Rocky Vista University College of Osteopathic Medicine	DO	2012
Connecticut	The Frank H. Netter MD School of Medicine at Quinnipiac University	MD	2013
Connecticut	University of Connecticut School of Medicine	MD	1961
Connecticut	Yale University School of Medicine	MD	1814
District of Colombia	George Washington University School of Medicine and Health Sciences	MD	1826
District of Colombia	Georgetown University School of Medicine	MD	1852

District of Colombia	Howard University College of Medicine	MD	1891
Florida	Florida International University Herbert Wertheim College of Medicine	MD	2009
Florida	Florida Atlantic University Charles E. Schmidt College of Medicine	MD	2011
Florida	Florida State University College of Medicine	MD	2000
Florida	The University of Miami Miller School of Medicine	MD	1952
Florida	University of South Florida Health Morsani College of Medicine	MD	1971
Florida	University of Central Florida College of Medicine	MD	2009
Florida	University of Florida College of Medicine	MD	1956
Florida	Lake Erie College of Osteopathic Medicine	DO	2008
Florida	Nova Southeastern College of Osteopathic Medicine	DO	1985
Georgia	Emory University School of Medicine	MD	1915
Georgia	Medical College of Georgia School of Medicine	MD	1833
Georgia	Mercer University School of Medicine	MD	1982
Georgia	Morehouse School of Medicine	MD	1975
Georgia	Philadelphia College of Osteopathic Medicine – Georgia Campus	DO	2009

Hawaii	University of Hawaii John A. Burns School of Medicine	MD	1973
Illinois	Chicago Medical School at Rosalind Franklin University of Medicine and Science	MD	1915
Illinois	Loyola University Chicago Stritch School of Medicine	MD	1915
Illinois	Northwestern University The Feinberg School of Medicine	MD	1860
Illinois	Rush Medical College of Rush University	MD	1844
Illinois	Southern Illinois University School of Medicine	MD	1970
Illinois	University of Chicago The Pritzker School of Medicine	MD	1927
Illinois	University of Illinois College of Medicine	MD	1883
Illinois	Midwestern University Chicago College of Osteopathic Medicine	DO	1900
Indiana	Indiana University School of Medicine	MD	1908
Indiana	Marian University College of Osteopathic Medicine	DO	2013
Iowa	University of Iowa Roy J. and Lucille A. Carver College of Medicine	MD	1871
Iowa	Des Moines University College of Osteopathic Medicine	DO	1898
Kansas	University of Kansas School of Medicine	MD	1906
Kentucky	University of Kentucky College of Medicine	MD	1960

Kentucky	University of Louisville School of Medicine	MD	1838
Kentucky	University of Pikeville Kentucky College of Osteopathic Medicine	DO	2001
Louisiana	Louisiana State University Health Sciences Center School of Medicine	MD	1969
Louisiana	Louisiana State University School of Medicine in New Orleans	MD	1931
Louisiana	Tulane University School of Medicine	MD	1835
Maine	University of New England College of Osteopathic Medicine	DO	1982
Maryland	Johns Hopkins University School of Medicine	MD	1897
Maryland	Uniformed Services University of the Health Sciences F. Edward Hebert School of Medicine	MD	1972
Maryland	University of Maryland School of Medicine	MD	1810
Massachusetts	Boston University School of Medicine	MD	1848
Massachusetts	Harvard Medical School	MD	1788
Massachusetts	Tufts University School of Medicine	MD	1894
Massachusetts	University of Massachusetts Medical School	MD	1962
Michigan	Central Michigan University College of Medicine	MD	2013

Michigan	Michigan State University College of Human Medicine	MD	1964
Michigan	Oakland University William Beaumont School of Medicine	MD	2011
Michigan	University of Michigan Medical School	MD	1851
Michigan	Wayne State University School of Medicine	MD	1869
Michigan	Michigan State University College of Osteopathic Medicine	DO	1969
Minnesota	Mayo Medical School	MD	1972
Minnesota	University of Minnesota Medical School	MD	1889
Mississippi	University of Mississippi School of Medicine	MD	1903
Mississippi	William Carey University College of Osteopathic Medicine	DO	2014
Missouri	Saint Louis University School of Medicine	MD	1902
Missouri	University of Missouri – Columbia School of Medicine	MD	1846
Missouri	University of Missouri – Kansas City School of Medicine	MD	1971
Missouri	Washington University in St. Louis School of Medicine	MD	1891
Missouri	A.T. Still University Kirksville College of Osteopathic Medicine	DO	1892
Missouri	Kansas City University of Medicine and Biosciences College of Osteopathic Medicine	DO	1916

Nebraska	Creighton University School of Medicine	MD	1893
Nebraska	University of Nebraska College of Medicine	MD	1882
Nevada	Touro University Nevada College of Osteopathic Medicine	DO	2008
Nevada	University of Nevada School of Medicine	MD	1967
New Hampshire	Geisel School of Medicine at Dartmouth	MD	1798
New Jersey	Cooper Medical School at Rowan University	MD	2012
New Jersey	University of Medicine and Dentistry of New Jersey – New Jersey Medical School	MD	1954
New Jersey	University of Medicine and Dentistry of New Jersey – Robert Wood Johnson Medical School	MD	1961
New Jersey	University of Medicine and Dentistry of New Jersey – School of Osteopathic Medicine	DO	1981
New Mexico	University of New Mexico School of Medicine	MD	1961
New York	Albany Medical College	MD	1839
New York	Albert Einstein College of Medicine of Yeshiva University	MD	1955
New York	Columbia University College of Physicians and Surgeons	MD	1769
New York	Hofstra University North Shore–LIJ School of Medicine	MD	2011

New York	Joan & Sanford I. Weill Medical College of Cornell University	MD	1899
New York	Mount Sinai School of Medicine of New York University	MD	1963
New York	New York Medical College	MD	1861
New York	New York University School of Medicine	MD	1842
New York	State University of New York Downstate Medical Center College of Medicine	MD	1860
New York	State University of New York Upstate Medical University	MD	1835
New York	Stony Brook University School of Medicine	MD	1971
New York	University at Buffalo State University of New York School of Medicine and Biomedical Sciences	MD	1847
New York	University of Rochester School of Medicine and Dentistry	MD	1925
New York	New York Institute of Technology New York College of Osteopathic Medicine	DO	1981
New York	Touro College of Osteopathic Medicine	MD	2011
North Carolina	Brody School of Medicine at East Carolina University	MD	1977
North Carolina	Duke University School of Medicine	MD	1930
North Carolina	University of North Carolina at Chapel Hill School of Medicine	MD	1879

North Carolina	Wake Forest School of Medicine of Wake Forest University Baptist Medical Center	MD	1902
North Carolina	Campbell University School of Osteopathic Medicine	DO	2013
North Dakota	University of North Dakota School of Medicine	MD	1905
Ohio	Case Western Reserve University School of Medicine	MD	1844
Ohio	Northeast Ohio Medical University	MD	1973
Ohio	The Ohio State University College of Medicine and Public Health	MD	1914
Ohio	The University of Toledo College of Medicine	MD	1964
Ohio	University of Cincinnati College of Medicine	MD	1821
Ohio	Wright State University Boonshoft School of Medicine	MD	1973
Ohio	Ohio University College of Osteopathic Medicine	DO	1980
Oklahoma	The University of Oklahoma College of Medicine	MD	
Oklahoma	Oklahoma State University Center for Health Sciences College of Osteopathic Medicine	DO	1978
Oregon	Oregon Health & Science University School of Medicine	MD	1888
Oregon	College of Osteopathic Medicine of the Pacific, Northwest	DO	2004

Pennsylvania	Drexel University College of Medicine	MD	1848
Pennsylvania	Jefferson Medical College of Thomas Jefferson University	MD	1826
Pennsylvania	Pennsylvania State University College of Medicine	MD	1963
Pennsylvania	Raymond and Ruth Perelman School of Medicine at the University of Pennsylvania	MD	1768
Pennsylvania	Temple University School of Medicine	MD	1904
Pennsylvania	The Commonwealth Medical College	MD	2008
Pennsylvania	University of Pittsburgh School of Medicine	MD	1887
Pennsylvania	Lake Erie College of Osteopathic Medicine	DO	1997
Pennsylvania	Philadelphia College of Osteopathic Medicine	DO	1899
Puerto Rico	Ponce School of Medicine	MD	1977
Puerto Rico	San Juan Bautista School of Medicine	MD	1978
Puerto Rico	Universidad Central del Caribe School of Medicine	MD	1976
Puerto Rico	University of Puerto Rico School of Medicine	MD	1950
Rhode Island	Warren Alpert Medical School of Brown University	MD	1814
South Carolina	Medical University of South Carolina College of Medicine	MD	1825
South Carolina	University of South Carolina School of Medicine	MD	1977

South Carolina	University of South Carolina School of Medicine Greenville	MD	2012
South Carolina	Virginia College of Osteopathic Medicine: Carolinas Campus	DO	2011
South Dakota	Sanford School of Medicine of the University of South Dakota	MD	1907
Tennessee	East Tennessee State University James H. Quillen College of Medicine	MD	1978
Tennessee	Meharry Medical College	MD	1877
Tennessee	University of Tennessee Health Science Center College of Medicine	MD	1911
Tennessee	Vanderbilt University School of Medicine	MD	1875
Tennessee	Lincoln Memorial University DeBusk College of Osteopathic Medicine	DO	2007
Texas	Baylor College of Medicine	MD	1901
Texas	Texas A&M Health Science Center College of Medicine	MD	1977
Texas	Texas Tech University Health Sciences Center Paul L. Foster School of Medicine (El Paso)	MD	2008
Texas	Texas Tech University Health Sciences Center School of Medicine	MD	1969
Texas	University of Texas Medical Branch at Galveston	MD	1892
Texas	University of Texas Medical School at Houston	MD	1972
Texas	University of Texas Medical School at San Antonio	MD	1959

Texas	University of Texas Southwestern Medical School at Dallas	MD	1943
Texas	University of North Texas Health Science Center at Fort Worth Texas College of Osteopathic Medicine	DO	1974
Utah	University of Utah School of Medicine	MD	1906
Vermont	University of Vermont College of Medicine	MD	1823
Virginia	Eastern Virginia Medical School	MD	1973
Virginia	University of Virginia School of Medicine	MD	1828
Virginia	Virginia Commonwealth University School of Medicine	MD	1839
Virginia	Virginia Tech Carilion School of Medicine	MD	2010
Virginia	Edward Via Virginia College of Osteopathic Medicine	DO	2007
Washington	University of Washington School of Medicine	MD	1946
Washington	Pacific Northwest University of Health Sciences	DO	2012
West Virginia	Marshall University Joan C. Edwards School of Medicine	MD	1977
West Virginia	West Virginia University School of Medicine	MD	1902
West Virginia	West Virginia School of Osteopathic Medicine	DO	1978
Wisconsin	Medical College of Wisconsin	MD	1913
Wisconsin	University of Wisconsin Medical School	MD	1907

The table above lists the MD and DO options in the US. Dual degrees, such as MD/PhD, MD/MBA, MD/JD, MD/MPH, and MD/MPP also exist. Do your research. Flip through the MSAR to learn all of your options and how to strategize which schools to include on your application list.

AMCAS Section VIII: Essays

Your medical school admissions story will coalesce in the personal comments essay, or personal statement. In this essay, you are asked to consider the following questions:

- Why have you selected the field of medicine?
- What motivates you to learn more about the field of medicine?
- What information do you want medical schools to know about you that has not been disclosed in another section of the application?

You have 5300 characters (about one page) to tell the admissions committee why you want to be a physician and why you will be an outstanding one. This, literally, is your admissions story. Tyler, Kevin, Padma, Mary, and Gabbi are back to show us how this is done.

When you read through these examples, remember all identifying information has been removed. In your personal comments essay, be specific.

Personal Statement Example 1: Tyler

Junior in large public university inspired by grandfather's 40-year career as family practitioner who confirmed importance of medicine's personal side through serving as EMT, Big Brother, and clinical research assistant.

Look how Tyler uses good essay writing techniques to tell his story. He starts with a "hook" to draw the reader in and set the essay's theme, follows with three supporting paragraphs, and concludes strongly. But this is not a cookie cutter personal statement merely repeating the work/activities section. Why? Because Tyler weaves the theme of building strong relationships with patients into every part of the essay.

"Physicians and patients alike will never forget your ever-lasting smile and upbeat spirit during your tenure here. You have meant so much to all of us and we want to thank you for everything." Piles of letters expressing the same sentiment started to accumulate on Dr. Clifford Seidel's desk. Suffering from advanced Alzheimer's, he sadly had little comprehension of the notes that poured in thanking him for over forty years of service. As I sat reading through the heart-felt letters of gratitude for Dr. Seidel, my "Grandpa Cliff," I noticed they all focused as much on his character as his medical prowess. He loved to tell me, "Physicians are not just in the medical business, they are in the people business." I want to be in this medical profession.

I began my medical journey as an eager EMT. Although I had years of advanced science and math courses to my credit, I had little medical knowledge. I realized it was important to determine if

I could use my aptitude and also face the human side of medicine. During rotations, I assisted on multiple traumas and received commendation from supervising paramedics. On one of my first few days in the Emergency Department (ED), a hectic afternoon with multiple traumas, the busy attending physician tasked me with checking patients' vitals, including monitoring the airway status of an elderly woman named Lucy. She had suffered an allergic reaction to her blood pressure medicine and required close monitoring. During her ED stay, Lucy did not have a single visitor, but I kept her distracted with several jokes to try to maintain a positive spirit and reduce her stress level. Upon discharge, I wheeled her to the car and she turned to say, "Thank you Hudson. I was very scared and alone today and you helped me through it." While I could not diagnose or medically treat her condition, I was able to provide the equally important side of complete medicine, my personal attention.

Serving in Big Brothers/Big Sisters taught me the importance of trust, confidentiality, and sincere interest, all of which will be integral parts of becoming an excellent physician. As the oldest of three children, being a big brother comes naturally, and I eagerly took on a new "little brother" named Neal. He started as a shy 12-year-old struggling to fit in. I looked for a connection we could share to bring him out of his shell and realized we both loved basketball. Neal informed me he loved to watch basketball, but no one had been around to teach him how to play. Our friendship grew with each jump shot as we learned about each other over games of "H-O-R-S-E." Over the next couple of years, while Neal's basketball game improved, he also began to flourish both socially and academically. As I entered my last week as Neal's big brother, he excelled in advanced math courses and played on the A basketball team. It was hard to tell Neal goodbye, as in fact I had grown as much as he had.

Even while assisting in clinical research, I realized how medicine is as much about the person as it is about the science. My research with Dr. Callahan started with a seemingly insurmountable stack of charts and empty Excel spreadsheets designed to map patient progress. As I monitored each patient's chart, I became enthralled in the story of each individual improvement. The majority of these patients were unable to complete daily tasks without significant pain. Yet, one year after surgery, most patients were walking without discomfort and able to resume the majority of daily activities. During one chart review, I read a letter reminding me of Grandpa Cliff. The patient had left a note relating how the surgery had completely changed his life stating, "Dr. Callahan...you have given me my life back, and I am forever grateful." Dr. Callahan had used his extensive training and innovative procedure to repair the patient's diseased hip and thereby changed this patient's quality of life in ways he may never fully witness. Doing the same for my patients is one of my greatest desires.

Following in the footsteps of Grandpa Cliff, I have learned my passion for medicine stems from both a fascination with the sciences and a love of people. During my undergraduate experience, I enjoyed and excelled in pre-medical courses. The sciences are my comfort zone, where I can excel and feel great accomplishment, and yet, it is the patient dynamic of medicine that has inspired me to pursue a medical career. I am aware physicians experience an inevitable spectrum of results in treating patients, and I know not every outcome will be ideal. I may see as much tragedy as joy. I, however, aspire to provide the greatest expertise and compassion to my patients as we partner together to provide the highest quality care.

Personal Statement Example 2: Kevin

Forty-year-old software developer returned to pre-med post-baccalaureate courses after caring for friends dying of AIDS and subsequently worked as HIV counselor, developed software for free clinic, and performed psychiatric research. He hopes to become internist or psychiatrist working with patients suffering from chronic disease.

How does a 40-year-old nontraditional candidate condense over twenty years of undergraduate and post-graduate life into one page and effectively convince admissions committees why he is leaving a lucrative career to be a physician? Read below to find out.

Shifting in his chair, chattering about the warm weather, and avoiding eye contact, the man across from me exuded anxiety. I did not know why Ben had come to a HIV counselor, but I realized direct questioning would not help me find out. I started by addressing the present moment and that he seemed anxious. As we chatted, Ben turned toward me, slowed his speech, and looked me in the eye, revealing that he may have exposed his partner to HIV. After we made a connection and discussed the options, Ben left the counseling session with a cautious resolve to talk frankly with his partner. This counseling interaction exemplifies qualities I will bring to the practice of medicine: the ability to build trust, to respond to people on their own terms, and to see patients as situated in biological, psychological, and cultural contexts.

I learned respect for different cultures from my mother, a school principal who moved us overseas after my father died. While in Central Asia, my mother arranged for a religious ceremony to honor the deity local residents believed lived in trees prior to having a tree removed from school property. Through such actions my mother taught me the importance of interacting with people from other cultures in terms consistent with their worldview.

While my childhood overseas provided invaluable lessons about respecting different cultures, moving almost yearly proved difficult given my natural shyness. I longed to be a real American kid, watching TV and drinking milk from a carton instead of the powdered version in Central Asia and Africa. When we returned to the United States, however, I initially felt lost in American culture. My extreme shyness and sense of dislocation increased in high school and college, leading to social challenges. My academic record reflects my distraction during those years. Despite fitful attempts to finish my degree, I left school to work as a computer programmer, which satisfied my analytic interests but did little to address my isolation.

In the 1990s, the AIDS epidemic refocused my attention on others. Before anti-retroviral combination therapy revolutionized HIV treatment, I cared for several friends dying of AIDS. Though initially terrified of David's thin, ashen body and blind eyes ravaged by CMV, I found a deep sense of peace and clarity helping him maintain his dignity as he became increasingly disabled. Interpreting the wishes of my friend David was difficult because dementia clouded his mind and an esophageal fungal infection inhibited his speech. But with the guidance of his expressive eyes, I learned that small gestures, such as soothing his lips with Vaseline or reading a chapter from Pinocchio, comforted him while he was dying. The opportunity to care for friends triggered self-exploration and led me to successfully obtain help for my own social anxiety. Healthy and focused, I decided to finish my undergraduate degree. Longing to study new ways of thinking, I majored in philosophy and felt drawn to thinkers who assert a meaningful life arises from concrete, bodily interaction with other human beings, rather than from isolated, detached reasoning.

To explore connections between body and mind, I volunteered as a research assistant in a Bay Area college's Psychophysiology and Social Interaction Laboratory. There I studied the physiological effects of induced emotions. I also observed dramatic physiological changes in couples during stressful conversations, again demonstrating that an individual's health greatly depends on context – in this case, the context of long-term, intimate relationships.

While finishing school, I reflected upon my satisfaction caring for sick friends, fascination with contextual understanding of human interactions, and lifelong interest in problem solving. I realized medicine is my calling and immediately set out to gain clinical experience. In addition to working as a HIV counselor, I volunteered as a clinic assistant at an urban community center serving immigrants. There, the trust of a Cantonese teenager who extended her arm for a flu shot reminded me of the fulfillment gained while caring for sick friends. Seeing patients suffer from diabetes because their diet dramatically changed reinforced my sense that health depends on social context. Repeatedly calling social service agencies to help an elderly Guatemalan woman find temporary housing heightened my resolve to use analytic skills to bring systematic change to service delivery and triggered my development of a system providing clinic patients with health education materials and case management services.

I am drawn to medicine because, uniquely among the care-giving professions, medicine has the ability to address patients as biological, social, and cultural beings. My varied experiences, including growing up overseas, caring for friends dying of AIDS, working as a HIV counselor, and assisting underserved immigrants, have all reinforced that understanding a patient's context is critical to providing appropriate care. As a physician, I will use this knowledge to help people develop their health in accordance with what gives their lives meaning.

Personal Statement Example 3: Padma

First generation Sri Lankan who became interested in ophthalmology as a child requiring glasses and pursued interest through participating in free eye clinics for disadvantaged inner city populations, performing ophthalmology research, and founding sustainable eye clinic in Sri Lanka.

You do not have to choose a medical specialty, such as internal medicine or surgery, upon applying to medical school. But if you have a passion for a certain part of medicine, explored through research, community service, extracurricular, or clinical activities, then it is appropriate to make this specialty part of your essay's theme. See how Padma starts with an excellent hook drawing the reader in (a theme I hope you notice in all of the essays), and then lays out an excellent thesis (last sentence of first paragraph) to set up the rest of the piece. She follows with four supporting paragraphs, which all relate back to the thesis, and finishes with a strong conclusion.

"Hey, Four-Eyes! Watch out for the ball!" Before I could look up from my weathered copy of Charlotte's Web, a red dodge ball hit me square in the face. I looked down as shards of glass lay scattered on the ground – my guide to the outside world destroyed in an instant. I felt frustrated that I was the first student in Mrs. Morrison's third grade class to need glasses and often asked my parents why this was the case. They suggested I borrow books from the school library to learn more about the fascinating science of sight. Over time, I began to view my need for glasses as a blessing in disguise. This early experience introduced me to the thrill of discovering knowledge and ignited a passion for vision that has lasted long after the books were due. After exploring the world of eyesight as a bench researcher, community vision screener, overseas volunteer, and clinic founder, I am confident serving as a physician will allow me to combine my dual passions for research and public health while drawing upon the skills gained from a sustained commitment to ophthalmology.

Pursuing multiple research opportunities in college allowed me to continue seeking answers to my own questions, while providing the freedom to think creatively and test the limits of current scientific understanding. During my three years in an ophthalmology lab, we investigated the potential for gene therapy to treat blind patients who suffered from inherited retinal disease. As a recipient of the University Scholars Scholarship, I completed a senior thesis analyzing the precise anatomical changes in the retina of a mouse model for Leber's Congenital Amaurosis (LCA). The results of my study identified benchmark values that can be used when assessing the efficacy of new treatments for LCA in mouse models.

Outside of the laboratory, I wanted to learn how research findings could be practically applied to improve health outcomes. I volunteered with a non-profit dedicated to improving sight for underprivileged communities and provided preliminary vision screenings at local health fairs. As community advocates, we relied on evidence-based interventions to engage and educate individuals who lacked access to vision services. Furthermore, we referred these individuals to other free national eye-coverage programs, thereby ensuring their continued vision care.

I then sought to gain a greater understanding of global health concerns by volunteering with the same non-profit in India. In a dusty village 20 miles from the state capital, a large crowd of men, women, children, goats, and cows stared back at us with mutual fascination. We screened hundreds of people for vision problems ranging from childhood refractive errors to adult macular degeneration. I noticed Swapna, whose warm mahogany skin glowed in stark contrast to her icy blue eyes. I soon realized her blue eyes stemmed not from genetics, but from cataracts resulting in near-blindness. We took Swapna back to the capital, and the next day she received cataract surgery. Within minutes, the ophthalmologist had replaced her opaque lens with a new artificial one. A few days later, Swapna's grandson clung to her paisley sari as a doctor removed the eye patch. While I could not understand the native tongue, I could feel Swapna's happiness as she conversed with the grandchild to whom she had often spoken, yet had never seen. She smiled while touching the boy's eyes, nose, and mouth, as if trying to translate his face into a new language. I was moved by the ophthalmologist's use of simple yet sophisticated methods to radically improve an individual's quality of life.

Inspired by my India experience, I felt compelled to act after learning of Sri Lanka's alarmingly high prevalence of untreated diabetic retinopathy. I proposed a clinic model to provide a complete screening for diabetic retinopathy at no cost to the patient. I relished the challenge to incorporate international standards of care while ensuring the program remained relevant to Sri Lanka's unique cultural context. I became acutely aware of the complexities of modern healthcare delivery as we delicately balanced the desire to provide the best quality of care with real-world constraints, such as rising medical costs and patient compliance obstacles. Undeterred by physicians' initial hesitation to work with someone so young, I successfully harnessed the skills and talents of numerous doctors in order to create an efficient method of screening and caring for diabetic patients and their families.

Each of my clinical experiences has demonstrated the importance of timely public health interventions to improving population health. As these experiences have been largely independent ventures based on my own initiative, I will adopt a more structured approach to furthering my understanding of health policies and practices by enrolling in the Master's of Public Health program in England this fall. Upon completing the MPH, I look forward to entering medical school and continuing my pursuit of a medical career dedicated to making a tangible impact on the lives of individual patients and underserved communities in the United States and abroad.

Personal Statement Example 4: Mary

MD/PhD candidate whose interest in research started while teaching music to autistic child and who used patience, thoughtful reflection, and communication skills practiced as singer to advance scientific investigations.

Mary, as a MD/PhD candidate, is required to write three essays – the personal statement and two further essays focused on research. Notice how Mary, though obviously gifted in research, uses her admissions narrative to prove how she will be both an excellent clinical physician and researcher.

She can sit at the piano for an hour, stroking the keys with deliberate intensity. Although Sarah cannot verbalize it, her love of music is unmistakable. As a member of Autism Partners volunteers, I am privileged to spend the afternoon with my "little partner" every other Saturday. Compared to a neurotypical seven year old, Sarah is delayed in motor skills, language, and social interaction, yet she has astounding musical talent. When I play notes, she plays back, carefully selecting tones that harmonize with mine. Music is an instrumental force in both of our lives. For Sarah, music is a means of communication. For me, music has been a guide in the progression of my career goals and the foundation from which I developed a desire to become a physician-scientist.

The musical experience that led me to medicine occurred in December 2001, as I performed with my high school Madrigal Singers at the first public reopening of the White House following September 11th. Our audience consisted of families of New York firefighters who had lost their lives in the World Trade Center attacks. This performance went beyond entertainment to become a consolation for grieving parents and spouses, and its healing power inspired me to help others in pain. In reflection, this occasion brought my medical career goal into clear focus and motivated me to pursue health-related research and clinical experiences.

In college my goal was decidedly a career in medicine, yet I did not abandon music. In fact, I found I could apply aspects of musical training, such as patience and thoughtful expression, to discussions with patients during my clinical research at University Hospital. Initially, interviewing patients post-operatively to document pain and activity levels was difficult. Visiting patients with merely the prescribed checklist often resulted in brief and strained responses. However, an open conversation with an elderly interviewee showed me there is an art to connecting with patients. After sharing experiences as a military wife and proud grandmother, she eagerly answered the questionnaire, and then added with a wink, "Maybe you'd like to meet my grandson." From this memorable dialogue, I realized talking with patients is not purely quantitative. Just as I trained to express music effectively to an audience, I began connecting with patients through emotion and reflection. The more I interacted with patients, the more curious I became about the inner workings of the body.

As a college senior, I joined an ovarian physiology lab and was captivated with investigating the underpinnings of infertility by exploring energy requirements of luteinizing granulosa cells. Discussion dominated our lab group, and my research mentor inspired me to ask questions and explore ideas. Even in the analytical field of molecular biology, musical training guided me. To my surprise, formulating hypotheses in science was similar to predicting harmonies in music; both skills required pattern analysis, insight, and creativity. As the songwriter and musical director of my college *a cappella* group, I learned to synthesize large amounts of detailed information, and this expertise directly applied to scientific experimentation. Biomedical research excited and challenged me in a way nothing had before. Convinced research was essential to understanding human biology and treating disease, I had to experience more.

For the past three years, research has been my focus. As a master's student investigating the role of RNA processing proteins in telomere maintenance, I became increasingly interested in relating my findings to clinical applications. Currently, as a National Institutes of Health research fellow, I explore axonal gene expression in developing sympathetic neurons with the desire to continue in the field of developmental neuroscience. However, research alone cannot treat patients. Only medical training will prepare me to heal and provide care. First drawn to medicine and later fascinated by research, I now know my talents and aspirations lie in both disciplines. MD/PhD training will help me to acquire the diverse skills needed to recognize relevant clinical questions, address them at the basic science level, and translate my findings back to the clinic.

At Autism Partners' final session of the school year, big and little partners joined for circle time. As the closing song commenced, a new voice resonated throughout the gym. It was Sarah, who loudly sang the first line of "Goodbye Partners." Tears formed in the program director's eyes. It was the first time we had ever heard her sing. With Sarah, I felt the power of human interaction, and the progress she has made through our musical connection embodies my motivation to become a physician. Yet I know that Sarah is not healed by music alone. It is through a combination of medical therapies, rooted in basic science research, that Sarah and other "little partners" will be fully empowered. I pursue the path of a physician-scientist to discover, heal, and empower.

Personal Statement Example 5: Gabbi

African-American woman who attended traditionally black college, served in sorority and club leadership roles, worked in free clinic serving indigent minority patients, and wants to become primary care physician focusing on decreasing health disparities in black communities.

Sometimes pre-meds from minority or other disadvantaged backgrounds feel it is necessary to hide their race/ethnicity, economic status, or familial issues from admissions committees. There is no need to hide from or be ashamed of who you are and where you come from. Gabbi does the opposite of concealing her background by using race as the center of her admissions narrative. So effective is Gabbi's story and overall application, she receives acceptance to numerous top 10 medical schools including Harvard.

During a Summer Medical and Dental Educational Program (SM-DEP) lecture on health disparities, I could not contain my disbelief and disappointment. Most of the statistics discussed had African Americans – those of my race – at the lowest end of the health spectrum. HIV/AIDS, diabetes, heart disease, stroke, and even cancer seem to affect my race more than others. We also learned about the reasons for these disparities, which include high-stress environments, lack of access to and poor quality of care, and minimal representation in the health care field. Many experiences have strengthened my lifelong dream of becoming a physician, but that lecture was the most meaningful. Afterwards, I knew I had a personal responsibility to reduce the disparities in my community by becoming an excellent physician. My research, clinical experiences, and time as a resident assistant have solidified my desire to become a physician who will focus on needs of the African American community by providing exceptional healthcare and health education.

In order to better understand how environmental stress may be a contributing factor to health disparities, I currently work with the psychology department at my university to research the correlation between psychological and physiological stress in the African American population. In the study "Cardiac Components of Anxiety," participants take a timed math test to show the functioning of the sympathetic nervous system and a stroop task to show parasympathetic functioning while we record heart rate variability. Abnormal heart rate variability has been correlated with common negative health outcomes in the African American community, and analysis of this data will show how stress affects heart rate variability in the sample population. Therefore, in the future, we may be able to see if coping mechanisms for stress can help to stabilize heart rate variability and prevent health issues. Both the one-on-one interaction with test participants and investigation of disease causes in my community have strengthened my passion to become a physician.

In addition to research, clinical experiences have confirmed my desire to become a physician. Because of my interest in pediatrics, I shadowed Dr. Baily Lovette at Washington Pediatric Hospital, which provides care to an underserved population. I watched as she examined the children's symptoms, made diagnoses, and designed treatment plans. She was also a great educator to parents, explaining her rationales and sympathetically addressing their concerns. One of her memorable patients had severe neurological issues due to complications from a vaccine, and whenever her family would come with concerns, Dr. Lovette greeted them warmly and answered all of their questions with compassion. During my time with Dr. Lovette, I saw how the basics of what doctors do – diagnose and treat disease – is connected to education. I am determined to be a doctor who provides excellent healthcare, which has a necessary element of educating patients and families about health and disease.

The importance of health education did not only manifest itself in clinical experience, but also in leadership opportunities. As a resident assistant for a hall comprised mostly of African-American freshman girls, I played a role akin to big sister. One day, a resident told me our floor had a pregnancy and a case of herpes. In response, I organized a sexual health program with the university student health center for my residents. An expert discussed the high rates of sexually transmitted infections (STIs) in our geographic area – especially among African American women – and methods for women to prevent pregnancy and STIs. Through this experience, I not only gained an interest in women's health, but also learned even more about the importance of leadership and health education.

My goal of becoming a physician stems from my desire to address health disparities, provide excellent healthcare and health education, and lead my community towards better health. I will take on health disparities in my community by understanding the contributing factors of disease, while providing the quality care many in this community are not able to receive. Like Dr. Lovette, I will diagnose and treat my patients while providing education about health and disease. Because I understand the role of leadership in health education, I will work to ensure my patients understand how health disparities affect them, which should empower them to maintain good health. I am only one person and cannot solve all of the problems of the African-American community on my own, but I know I will be a physician who makes a change with the people who I treat and teach.

AMCAS Section IX: Standardized Tests

In this section, you will input your MCAT score(s). Applicants to combined programs who request other scores, such as Graduate Management Admissions Test (GMAT), Law School Admissions Test (LSAT), or Graduate Records Examination (GRE) can also submit these scores in the standardized tests section.

Not Quite The End

Congratulations! You made it to the end of the AMCAS application and the Six Buckets. Though you may feel overwhelmed by the pre-med requirements, understanding what is expected of you provides a distinct advantage when navigating the competitive process of becoming a physician. Hopefully, this book has clarified the complexity of how to be pre-med and will help you make good life choices while preparing for a medical career. Further, you have now learned to avoid "checking the boxes," to instead do what you love because then you will likely do it well, and to create a compelling story for medical school admissions.

Submitting the AMCAS application does not end the medical school admissions process. After completing the primary application, medical schools require you answer secondary application essays and attend interviews. Subsequently, post-interview strategy, such as sending update letters or a letter of intent, may help you gain acceptance. Though time consuming, these extra application steps provide further opportunities to tell your story. Details on these aspects of the medical school application will be of concern nearer to when you apply and are explained thoroughly in the latest edition of *The Medical School Admissions Guide.*

The road to doctorhood is filled with hurdles. But every pre-med obstacle can be leapt gracefully with thoughtful advanced planning, appropriate strategy, and practice. In the future, I hope you reflect on the pre-med journey as a time of optimism, curiosity, and excitement and find the years of hard work pay off the minute you help your first patient.

MYTH BUSTERS: APPLICATION SKILLS
The pre-med rumor mill has created the following myths. All of these myths have been busted.

- Medical school has one of the easiest applications of all graduate schools.
- Applying soon after the AMCAS opens in June offers no advantage in the application process.
- Courses taken abroad don't have to be listed on the medical school application.
- All fifteen AMCAS work/activities must be filled.
- The personal statement is rarely read and has little weight in the medical school application.
- Once you have completed the AMCAS application, the medical school application process is complete.

FILL IT UP

Use the area below to take notes on filling
the Application Skills Bucket

If You Found This Book Helpful...

...you may also enjoy these other best-selling books and medical school admissions resources by Dr. Miller:

The Medical School Admissions Guide: A Harvard MD's Week-by-Week Admissions Handbook, 2nd Edition

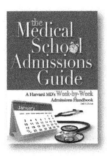

Available at amazon.com, barnesandnoble.com, and MDadmit.com
Updated regularly, so be sure to look for most recent edition

How To Get Into Medical School With A Low GPA

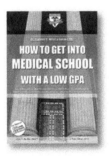

Available at www.howtobepremed.com
Enter coupon code "Accepted!" for $20 off cover price

MDadmit Medical School Admissions Bootcamps

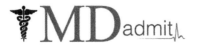

Sign up at MDadmit.com

About the Author

D r. Suzanne M. Miller was raised near Washington, DC and studied history and science at Harvard College. While attending Harvard Medical School, she began admissions consulting as a Pre-Medical Tutor and then Co-Chair of the Eliot House Pre-Medical Committee. After receiving her MD, she trained at Stanford University in Emergency Medicine.

Dr. Miller now splits her time between Washington, DC and New York City working as an emergency physician and running MDadmit, a medical school admissions consulting service. She is proud to announce the start of MDadmit Medical School Admissions Bootcamps in 2013. Dr. Miller also enjoys teaching, traveling internationally, and serving as a physician for Racing the Planet adventure races, activities that have allowed her to make footprints on seven continents.

CPSIA information can be obtained
at www.ICGtesting.com
Printed in the USA
BVHW03s2047010618
517876BV00008B/196/P

9 781936 633555